# Peri-Operative Fluid Management

*Series editors* **Monty Mythen and Hugh Montgomery**

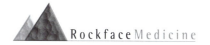

First published in Great Britain in 2007
by Rockface Medicine
PO Box 371
Reigate
RH2 2BH

Text © Rockface Medicine 2007

All rights reserved. No part of this publication may be reproduced, stored in a retrieval system, or transmitted, in any form or by any means, electronic, mechanical, photocopying, recording or otherwise, without prior written permission of the publisher and copyright owner, nor be otherwise circulated in any form of binding or cover other than that in which it is published and without a similar condition including this condition being imposed on the subsequent purchaser.

A CIP catalogue record for this book is available from the British Library

ISBN 978-0-9556126-0-2

Produced by Pagewise

*Art direction and coordination*
Mónica Bratt
monica.bratt@btinternet.com

Printed and bound in Great Britain
by Halstan and Co. Ltd

# Contents

*page*

5 **Foreword**
*Professor Sir Bruce E. Keogh*

7 **Introduction**

9 **Summary of Round Table Conclusions**
*Henrik Kehlet, T J Gan, Monty Mythen*

15 **Speakers Abstracts**

17 **Peri-operative fluid dynamics**
*Kathrine Holte*

25 **Goal directed fluid administration – peri-operative perspectives**
*T J Gan*

33 **Goal-directed fluid administration – ICU perspectives**
*Mike Grocott*

39 **Peri-operative volume management guided by venous or tissue oxygenation**
*Niels H. Secher*

47 **Peri-operative renal failure – a great fluid perspective**
*Tony Roche*

## Contents *continued*

- 59 **Peri-operative fluid management – bowel function / oral nutrition, fast-tracking and design issues**
  *Henrik Kehlet*

- 65 **Restricted fluid regimen and volumes of colloid / crystalloid**
  *Birgitte Brandstrup*

- 75 **Fluid therapy and coagulation**
  *Mike James*

- 93 **Interviews**

- 99 **Bibliography**

# Foreword

**It is increasingly recognised** that the choice of fluid administered to surgical patients may have a profound impact on their outcome. How much and what kind of fluid should we give, and when? Strong and differing views prevail, but what is the truth? Does saline cause an acidosis, and if it does is this necessarily a bad thing? Do starches in colloid cause renal failure? This short report summarises the best available evidence as reviewed by the leading world experts. As such, it is a valuable and timely contribution to the literature and to good patient care.

**Professor Sir Bruce E. Keogh**

*Professor of Cardiac Surgery*
*University College London*

# Introduction

**Good fluid management** is an essential component of good patient care. Poor intra-operative fluid management can cost a patient their life. This most fundamental of subjects remains highly controversial. In August 2006 a group of internationally recognised experts on intra-operative fluid management met in London, UK with the hope of reaching a consensus and creating a clear take-home message. The stated aim of the Round Table was:

- To tidy up the **language** of peri-operative fluid therapy.
- To summarise **best available evidence** and offer an intra-operative fluid management plan.
- To identify gaps in the literature and **propose future studies**.

This book and the disk that is available to accompany it present the *prime cuts* from that meeting in word, sound and vision.

Further material can also be found at www.rockfacemedicine.com. The key take-home message is:

**Individualised**
**Targeted**
**Fluid**
**Therapy**

# Summary of Round Table Conclusions

## Summary of round table conclusions
*2nd August 2006, London, UK*

Henrik Kehlet, TJ Gan, Monty Mythen

- Peri-operative fluid management is of fundamental importance. Poor peri-operative fluid management causes morbidity and mortality.

- It seems clear that in minor surgery 1-2 litres of Lactated Ringer's solution improves outcome.

- In intermediate surgery avoiding central hypovolaemia by the administration of 3 litres of Lactated Ringer's may also improve outcome although the benefits are less clear. From the blinded studies using a fast-track approach there is certainly no suggestion that larger volumes caused excess harm.

- The rest of this is about MAJOR surgery.

- Peri-opeartive fluid management is just one component of numerous factors that determine outcome as emphasised by the multi-modal approach to fast track surgery.

- There is inadequate education and knowledge on this important subject.

- There is an inadequate evidence base to inform evidence based recommendations.

- However, there is enough evidence from PCTs to guide better practice.

- The language that has been used in many peri-operative fluid management studies has been ill-defined and has created confusion. Terms like "liberal", "restricted" and "optimised" are commonly used to mean "avoid hypovolaemia" or avoid "fluid excess".

- It was agreed that "targeted fluid therapy" best defined the common objective.

- It was unanimously agreed that:

  - Hypovolaemia was not in the patient's best interest.

  - Fluid excess was also not in the patient's best interest.

  - It was important to try and understand/quantify deficits and replace with similar volumes and composition. Water with water, salts with salts, plasma with plasma, etc.

  - In most surgical cases water and electrolyte deficits can be effectively replaced with a balanced isotonic crystalloid (e.g. lactated Ringer's solution) rather than isotonic saline solution. Blood losses can be replaced with a colloid (e.g. hydroxyethyl starch) ideally suspended in a balanced electrolyte formulation that has a composition similar to human plasma. Higher blood losses will need to be replaced with red blood cells and blood products.

  - Intravascular volume status cannot be reliably determined using static pressure measurements (e.g. BP, CVP, PAOP). Flow measurements are better.

  - All major surgical cases should have their cardiac output measured.

# Summary of round table conclusions

- Central hypovolaemia is best avoided by giving colloid boluses with the aim of achieving maximum stroke volume.
- Ideal monitors of intravascular volume status and tissue perfusion remain unmet clinical needs.

## Studies proposed by the group

1 "Restricted" (i.e. Brandstrup study restricted group) vs "restricted" plus SV max with colloid.

2 Colloid vs crystalloid in trauma (pragmatic) – ongoing with Mike James in UCT, South Africa.

3 "Standard of care" vs SV max with colloid. Large multi-centre PCT in colonic surgery.

4 "Standard of care" vs fluid targeted to cerebral oxygen sats – main outcome = cognitive dysfunction.

5 Colloid vs crystalloid – max SV in both groups. Colonic surgery – with ethics at UCLH.

6 "Standard of care" vs colloid SV max in FAST TRACK colonic surgery.

7 Max SV with different fluids (HES, Gelo, NS and balanced) – renal dysfunction.

8 Colloid vs crystalloid in ambulatory surgery.

9 "Standard of care" vs max SV in elderly high risk surgery.

# Speakers' Abstracts

# Peri-operative fluid dynamics

# Kathrine Holte

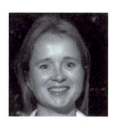

### Current position
Resident
Dept. of Surgical Gastroenterology
Hvidovre University Hospital
Copenhagen, Denmark

### Research fields
Fluid management
Surgical pathophysiology

### Current main research projects
We are conducting a series of randomized clinical studies with high vs low peri-operative fluid substitution in several surgical procedures (laparoscopic cholecystectomy, colonic surgery, orthopedic surgery) as well as experimental studies in volunteers to investigate the pathophysiology and clinical outcomes of various peri-operative fluid management strategies.

# Peri-operative fluid dynamics
Kathrine Holte

*Department of Surgical Gastroenterology*
*Hvidovre University Hospital*
*Copenhagen, Denmark*

The physiologic stress response to surgery induces inflammation, catabolism and fluid retention[1]. Vascular permeability is increased proportionately to the size of injury (surgery), inducing distribution of fluid from the intra-vascular to the interstitial space[1]. It was previously believed that surgery elicited an obligatory decrease in functional (i.e. exchangeable) ECV, findings since contradicted by others and attributed mainly to inadequacy in sampling techniques[2].

*Vascular permeability is increased proportionately to the size of injury (surgery)*

In volume kinetic analysis the distribution and elimination of an infused fluid volume, based on the fractional dilution of blood by measuring hemoglobin concentrations, is estimated by application of mathematical analysis[3]. The concept is based on the assumption that the body strives to maintain volume homeostasis of fluid spaces, in which an infused amount of fluid strives to maintain an ideal (target) volume, and leaves the occupied space at a rate proportional to the deviation from that target volume[3]. Infused crystalloid usually distribute to a central and a remote functional body fluid space, with sizes reasonably well correlating to the plasma and interstitial volumes[3,4]. The method has been proven effective in distinguishing normo-vs hypovolemic conditions as well as peri-operative fluid shifts. Elimination of infused crystalloid has been found significantly decreased during anesthesia[5] and surgery[6-8]. The method is exploratory and offers an alternative model to investigate internal fluid shifts and distribution and elimination of an intravenous fluid load. So what are the clinical implications and future research areas within peri-operative fluid dynamics and which outcomes should be measured?

*Elimination of infused crystalloid... decreased during anesthesia and surgery*

In *minor (ambulatory) surgery* it is well-documented that fluid substitution to correct preoperative dehydration (1-2 L vs. no fluid) may improve recovery[9-11]. In *medium-size procedures*, one recent randomized study found intra-operative administration of ~3 l compared to ~1 l Ringer's lactate reduced the cardiovascular hormonal responses, improved peri-operative organ functions, improved recovery and reduced hospital stay[12]. To further characterize the findings of this study we applied volume kinetic analysis with a fluid load of 12.5 ml kg$^{-1}$ RL infused pre- and 4 hours post-operatively with 15 ml kg$^{-1}$ vs. 40 ml kg$^{-1}$ RL administered intra-operatively in the same setting as described above[13]. We found that distribution and elimination of this fluid load was not altered by intra-operative fluid administration but it was eliminated slightly more rapidly after than before surgery. That fluid load was readily excreted regardless of intraoperative fluid administration indicates no significant dehydration or hypervolemia to be present. Further studies are currently set up to clarify the effects of crystalloid vs colloid management on volume kinetics in laparoscopic cholecystectomy and on volume kinetics after major surgical procedures.

In *major surgical procedures* both so-called "fluid restriction" and "goal-directed"/individualized fluid therapy has been found to improve outcome[14,15] (discussed in details by others). To further clarify effects of peri-operative fluid administration, studies on peri-operative physiology are needed. Recently, two such randomized clinical trials were conducted. In 48 patients undergoing knee arthroplasty, we found that a "liberal" (~ 4,3 l) vs. a "restrictive" (~1,7 l) peri-operative fluid regimen may lead to significant hypercoagulability and a reduction in vomiting but without differences in other recovery parameters or hospital stay[16]. And in 32 patients a "liberal" (~ 5 l) vs. a "restrictive" (~1,7 l) peri-operative fluid regimen may not deteriorate functional outcome after fast-track colonic surgery[17]. However, a "restrictive" fluid regimen without a sufficient pre- and early intra-operative volume load may predispose to increased morbidity as indicated by the finding of 3 anastomotic leakages in the "restrictive" group vs. 0 in the "liberal" group (although not a primary outcome)[17].

*There is a need for procedure-specific randomized clinical trials*

Regarding the type of fluid to be administered, we recently conducted a systematic review of 80 randomized trials in elective non-cardiac surgery, concluding that no conclusions on the administration of colloids vs crystalloids in elective surgery could be made with the presently available data, mainly due to lack of standardization and measurements of relevant clinical/physiological endpoints in the available literature[18].

In summary, in both intermediate and major surgery, there is a need for procedure-specific randomized clinical trials evaluating relevant functional physiologic outcome as well as large outcome studies evaluating morbidity/mortality with a fluid administration regimen designated to avoid both fluid excess and hypovolemia[19].

# Reference List

1 Holte K, Sharrock NE, Kehlet H. *Pathophysiology and clinical implications of peri-operative fluid excess.* Br J Anaesth 2002; 89: 622-32.

2 Brandstrup B, Svensen C, Engquist A. *Hemorrhage and operation cause a contraction of the extracellular space needing replacement evidence and implications? A systematic review.* Surgery 2006; 139: 419-32.

3 Hahn RG, Drobin D, Stahle L. *Volume kinetics of Ringer's solution in female volunteers.* Br J Anaesth 1997; 78: 144-8.

4 Svensen C, Hahn RG. *Volume kinetics of Ringer solution, dextran 70, and hypertonic saline in male volunteers.* Anesthesiology 1997; 87: 204-12.

5 Holte K, Foss NB, Svensen C, Lund C, Madsen JL, Kehlet H. *Epidural anesthesia, hypotension, and changes in intravascular volume.* Anesthesiology 2004; 100: 281-6.

6 Sjostrand F, Hahn RG. *Volume kinetics of glucose 2.5% solution during laparoscopic cholecystectomy.* Br J Anaesth 2004; 92: 485-92.

7 Ewaldsson CA, Hahn RG. *Kinetics and extravascular retention of acetated ringer's solution during isoflurane or propofol anesthesia for thyroid surgery.* Anesthesiology 2005; 103: 460-9.

8 Olsson J, Svensen CH, Hahn RG. *The volume kinetics of acetated Ringer's solution during laparoscopic cholecystectomy.* Anesthesia & Analgesia 2004; 99: 1854-60.

9 Holte K, Kehlet H. *Compensatory fluid administration for preoperative dehydration – does it improve outcome?* Acta Anaesthesiol Scand 2002; 46: 1089-93.

10 Maharaj CH, Kallam SR, Malik A, Hassett P, Grady D, Laffey JG. *Preoperative intravenous fluid therapy decreases postoperative nausea and pain in high risk patients.* Anesthesia & Analgesia 2005; 100: 675-82.

11 Ali SZ, Taguchi A, Holtmann B, Kurz A. *Effect of supplemental pre-operative fluid on postoperative nausea and vomiting.* Anaesthesia 2003; 58: 780-4.

12 Holte K, Klarskov B, Christensen DS, Lund C, Nielsen KG, Bie P, Kehlet H. *Liberal versus restrictive fluid administration to improve recovery after laparoscopic cholecystectomy: a randomized, double-blind study.* Ann Surg 2004; 240: 892-9.

13 Holte K, Hahn RG, Ravn L, Bertelsen KG, Hansen S, Kehlet H. *The influence of liberal vs restrictive intra-operative fluid management on the elimination of a postoperative intravenous fluid load* (submitted).

14 Brandstrup B, Tonnesen H, Beier-Holgersen R et al. *Effects of intra-venous fluid restriction on postoperative complications: comparison of two peri-operative fluid regimens: a randomized assessor-blinded multicenter trial.* Ann Surg 2003; 238: 641-8.

15 Grocott MP, Mythen MG, Gan TJ. *Peri-operative fluid management and clinical outcomes in adults.* Anesth Analg 2005; 100: 1093-106.

16 Holte K, Kristensen BB, Valentiner L, Foss NB, Husted H, Kehlet H. *Liberal vs restrictive fluid management in knee arthroplasty. A randomized, double-blind study* (submitted).

17 Holte K, Foss NB, Andersen J, Lund C, Valentiner L, Bie P, Kehlet H. *Liberal vs. restrictive fluid management in fast-track colonic surgery. A randomized, double-blind study* (submitted).

18 Holte K, Kehlet H. *Fluid therapy and surgical outcome in elective surgery – a need for reassessment in fast-track surgery – A systematic review.* J Am Coll Surg 2006; 202: 989.

19 Boldt J. *Fluid management of patients undergoing abdominal surgery – more questions than answers?* Eur J Anaesthesiol 2006; 23: 631-40.

# Goal-directed fluid administration
## – peri-operative perspectives

# T J Gan

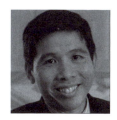

### Current position
Professor of Anesthesiology, Medical Director of the Duke Clinical Anesthesia Research Endeavor (CARE) and Senior Research Fellow at Duke Center for Integrative Medicine, Durham, NC, USA

Prof Gan has received the Society of Ambulatory Anesthesia Young Investigator Award, and the International Anesthesia Research Society (IARS) Clinical Scholar Research Award. He is a member of several professional organizations and serves on the Editorial Board of *Anesthesia*, *Acute Pain* and *Clinical Research*.

Prof Gan's widely published research includes: prevention of post-operative nausea and vomiting, fluid management during surgery and monitoring techniques, intravenous anesthesia and post-operative pain. He is the author or co-author of over 100 scientific articles in peer-reviewed medical journals and numerous abstracts, reviews and chapters published in medical textbooks.

# Goal-directed fluid administration – peri-operative perspectives
T J Gan

*Department of Anesthesiology*
*Duke University Medical Center*
*Durham, NC, USA*

Since the late 1950s a succession of authors have described an association between peri-operative cardiac output and survival following major surgery: the survivors exhibiting higher values than the non-survivors.[1-3] From these observations the hypothesis developed that using the cardiac output and oxygen delivery values exhibited by the survivors, as goals for all patients, would reduce overall mortality[1]. In 1988 Shoemaker et al[4] demonstrated that targeting specific values for cardiac index, oxygen delivery and oxygen consumption, using fluids and inotropes to achieve these goals, resulted in a reduction in mortality and morbidity.

Since then a number of single center randomized controlled trials have been conducted, the majority of which support this original positive result. Five studies have used the same hemodynamic goals as the original study by Shoemaker. Two of these were large (>100 patient) studies on high-risk general surgical and vascular patients and both demonstrated a statistically significant reduction in mortality in the protocol groups[5,6]. Two were studies of major trauma surgery and these were both conducted by the same group[7,8]. The first smaller study showed a trend towards reduction in mortality in the protocol group and this was confirmed by a statistically significant reduction in protocol group mortality in the second, larger trial. The fifth study in this group was a small trial focusing on surgery for hepatobiliary carcinoma and demonstrated a reduction in liver failure and hyperbilirubinemia although this was not their specified primary outcome variable[9]. An older study using a similar philosophy, but with less clearly defined goals, in patients undergoing hip fracture surgery also demonstrated a significant mortality reduction[10]. Somewhat different results have been obtained in a series of papers in which patients presenting for major vascular or aortic surgery were studied[11-13]. The goals for cardiac index and oxygen delivery used in these trials were significantly lower and the overall mortality for each trial was also low. These studies did not demonstrate a significant reduction in mortality, or in some cases complications, however in only one of these studies were there more deaths in the protocol than control groups[11].

Targeting mixed venous oxygen saturation (SvO2) as an indirect index of oxygen delivery has also been studied in two trials. The first patients studied had aortic or lower limb arterial surgery and failed to demonstrate a significant morbidity or mortality difference between control and protocol groups[14]. More recently a large Scandinavian study of patients undergoing elective coronary revascularization with cardiopulmonary bypass demonstrated a significant reduction in length of stay in those randomized to maintenance of SvO2 > 70% and lactate ≤ 2 mmol·L$^{-1}$ when compared with controls[15].

A number of published studies using intra-operative esophageal Doppler monitoring of cardiac output compared a stroke volume optimization algorithm with standard fluid management. In the first study patients with normal left ventricular function undergoing coronary artery revascularization had a statistically significant reduction in length of both ICU and overall hospital stay in the protocol group[16]. Subsequently, other investigators demonstrated a reduction in hospital length of stay in elderly patients having hip prosthesis surgery who were managed in the protocol group[17,18]. Gan and colleagues, in a study using a similar optimization algorithm, demonstrated a reduction in hospital stay and earlier return to tolerating solid food in the protocol group undergoing major non-cardiac surgery[19]. A more recent study reinforced the earlier findings[20]. Conway et al also demonstrated a lower incidence of ICU admission in the goal-directed fluid therapy group[21].

Spahn and Chassot in a recent editorial concluded that advanced monitoring alone is neither sufficient nor beneficial. Only combining monitoring with a clear management algorithm aiming at the optimization of the stroke volume with colloid boluses in the presence of a knowledgeable anesthesiologist will improve outcome of patients[22].

*combining monitoring with a clear management algorithm*

# Reference List

1 Shoemaker W C, Montgomery E S, Kaplan E, and Elwyn D H. *Physiological patterns in surviving and non-surviving shock patients. Use of sequential cardiorespiratory parameters in defining criteria for therapeutic goals and early warning of death.* Archives of Surgery 1973; 106: 630-6.

2 Boyd AR, Tremblay, R E, Spencer, F C, and Bahnson H T. *Estimation of Cardiac Output Soon After Cardiac Surgery With Cardiopulmonary Bypass.* Annals of Surgery 1959; 150: 613-25.

3 Clowes GaDG, LRM. *Circulatory Response to Trauma of Surgical Patients.* Metabolism 1960; 9: 67-81.

4 Shoemaker WC, Appel PL, Kram HB et al. *Prospective trial of supra-normal values of survivors as therapeutic goals in high-risk surgical patients.* Chest 1988; 94: 1176-86.

5 Boyd O, Grounds RM, Bennett ED. *A randomized clinical trial of the effect of deliberate peri-operative increase of oxygen delivery on mortality in high-risk surgical patients.* Jama 1993; 270: 2699-707.

6 Wilson J, Woods I, Fawcett J, et al. *Reducing the risk of major elective surgery: randomised controlled trial of peri-operative optimisation of oxygen delivery.* BMJ 1999; 318: 1099-103.

7 Fleming A, Bishop M, Shoemaker W et al. *Prospective trial of supra-normal values as goals of resuscitation in severe trauma.* Archives of Surgery 1992; 127: 1175-9; discussion 9-81.

8 Bishop MH, Shoemaker WC, Appel PL et al. *Prospective, randomized trial of survivor values of cardiac index, oxygen delivery, and oxygen consumption as resuscitation endpoints in severe trauma* [see comments]. Journal of Trauma-Injury Infection & Critical Care 1995; 38: 780-7.

9 Ueno S, Tanabe G, Yamada H, et al. *Response of patients with cirrhosis who have undergone partial hepatectomy to treatment*

*aimed at achieving supranormal oxygen delivery and consumption.* Surgery 1998; 123: 278-86.

10 Schultz RJ, Whitfield GF, LaMura JJ et al. *The role of physiologic monitoring in patients with fractures of the hip.* Journal of Trauma-Injury Infection & Critical Care 1985; 25: 309-16.

11 Bender JS, Smith-Meek MA, Jones CE. *Routine pulmonary artery catheterization does not reduce morbidity and mortality of elective vascular surgery: results of a prospective, randomized trial.* Annals of Surgery 1997; 226: 229-36; discussion 36-7.

12 Berlauk JF, Abrams JH, Gilmour IJ et al. *Preoperative optimization of cardiovascular hemodynamics improves outcome in peripheral vascular surgery. A prospective, randomized clinical trial* [see comments]. Annals of Surgery 1991; 214: 289-97; discussion 98-9.

13 Valentine RJ, Duke ML, Inman MH et al. *Effectiveness of pulmonary artery catheters in aortic surgery: a randomized trial.* Journal of Vascular Surgery 1998; 27: 203-11; discussion 11-2.

14 Ziegler DW, Wright JG, Choban PS, Flancbaum L. *A prospective randomized trial of preoperative "optimization" of cardiac function in patients undergoing elective peripheral vascular surgery* [see comments]. Surgery 1997; 122: 584-92.

15 Polonen P, Ruokonen E, Hippelainen M et al. *A prospective, randomized study of goal-oriented hemodynamic therapy in cardiac surgical patients.* Anesth Analg 2000; 90: 1052-9.

16 Mythen MG, Webb AR. *Peri-operative plasma volume expansion reduces the incidence of gut mucosal hypo perfusion during cardiac surgery.* Archives of Surgery 1995; 130: 423-9.

17 Sinclair S, James S, Singer M. *Intraoperative intravascular volume optimisation and length of hospital stay after repair of proximal femoral fracture: randomised controlled trial* [see comments]. BMJ 1997; 315: 909-12.

18 Venn R, Steele A, Richardson P et al. *Randomized controlled trial to*

*investigate influence of the fluid challenge on duration of hospital stay and peri-operative morbidity in patients with hip fractures.* Br J Anaesth 2002; 88: 65-71.

19 Gan TJ, Soppitt A, Maroof M et al. *Goal directed intraoperative fluid administration reduces length of hospital stay after major surgery.* Anesthesiology 2002; 97: 820-6.

20 Wakeling HG, McFall MR, Jenkins CS et al. *Intraoperative oesophageal Doppler guided fluid management shortens postoperative hospital stay after major bowel surgery.* British Journal of Anaesthesia 2005; 95: 634-42.

21 Critchley LA, Conway F. *Hypotension during subarachnoid anaesthesia: haemodynamic effects of colloid and metaraminol* [see comments]. Br J Anaesth 1996; 76: 734-6.

22 Spahn DR, Chassot P-G. CON: *Fluid restriction for cardiac patients during major noncardiac surgery should be replaced by goal-directed intravascular fluid administration.*[comment]. Anesth & Analg 2006; 102: 344-6.

# Goal-directed fluid administration
## – ICU perspectives

# Mike Grocott

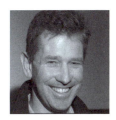

## Current position

Mike Grocott is a Senior Lecturer in Intensive Care Medicine at University College London (UCL) and honorary consultant anaesthetist at the Whittington Hospital and UCL Hospitals. He is co-director of the UCL Centre for Aviation Space and Extreme Environment Medicine, deputy director of the UCL Institute of Human Health and Performance and is an honorary lecturer in Physiology.

Mike is also director of Xtreme-Everest and was expedition leader of the Xtreme-Everest medical research expedition in spring 2007. His research interests include human responses to hypoxia, measuring and improving outcome following major surgery and fluid therapy.

# Goal-directed fluid administration – ICU perspectives
Mike Grocott

*Senior Lecturer*
*Intensive Care Medicine*
*UCL, London*

In the late 80s and early 90s several randomized controlled clinical studies demonstrated improved outcomes in the peri-operative setting using "optimization" or "goal-directed therapy"[1-3]. The intervention in these studies was the targeting of fluid and inotrope and vasodilator therapy at specific goals of oxygen delivery, oxygen consumption, cardiac output or mixed venous oxygen saturations. The studies tested Shoemaker's hypothesis that targeting the oxygen flux variables exhibited by survivors of high-risk major surgery in all patients would improve overall survival.

*targeting of fluid and inotrope and vasodilator therapy at specific goals*

A similar approach in the setting of established critical illness was tested in three studies in the 1990s. An RCT by Tuchschmidt did not show any benefit from a strategy aimed at elevating oxygen delivery in patients with septic shock[4]. Hayes then published an RCT showing an increased mortality in patients managed to specific oxygen delivery goals[5]. The following year Gattinoni published a multi-centre RCT which did not demonstrate any difference in outcomes between patients randomized to GDT aimed at increasing the cardiac index to a supranormal level or increasing mixed venous oxygen saturation to a normal level when compared with a control group[6].

More recently Rivers has demonstrated that in severe sepsis and septic shock the early institution of "goal-directed therapy" reduces mortality and improves other outcomes when tested in a randomized controlled clinical trials[7]. The Rivers GDT package consisted of fluids, blood and inotropes targeted towards raising the SvO2 >70%.

*"goal-directed therapy" reduces mortality and improves other outcomes*

*How do we interpret these apparently contradictory data?*

Firstly these are complex studies in different phases of critical illness, involving the use of a monitored variable to guide algorithms prescribing the administration of related but distinct interventions, to a variety of goals. Comparison between studies is difficult.

Secondly there is variation in the success of achievement of goals in the studies. Where goals are not achieved in the intervention group or where no differences in physiological end-points is demonstrated between the intervention and control groups, it is hard to interpret differences in outcome data whether these support efficacy for the intervention or not.

Thirdly the study by Rivers is the only study supporting the use of GDT in critical illness and this awaits replication. It is possible, although very unlikely, that the result of this study occurred by random chance and does not represent a true treatment effect.

Finally, and probably most importantly, when addressing the question "why are these types of intervention efficacious in one context (peri-operative setting) but not in an apparently similar one (critical illness)?" it is possible that the underlying pathophysiology of these clinical situations differs in such a way that there is a true difference in response to treatment.

A developing understanding of the metabolic responses associated with established critical illness supports this concept. Specifically Singer[8] and others have suggested that multiple organ failure is characterised by a reduction in cellular energetic activity analogous to a "hibernation" type response. This is in contrast to the response to acute injury which is characterized by a fight or flight response with increased oxygen consumption. It may be that treatment targeted at increasing oxygen delivery is efficacious in the setting of acute injury (peri-operative, trauma, early sepsis) when the natural physiological response is to maintain adequate oxygen delivery in the face of increased consumption. Conversely in established critical illness the body's response is to decrease oxygen utilization and perhaps increase the efficiency of oxygen metabolism. Therefore it may be that in this case therapies should be targeted at facilitating these processes and minimizing additional injury.

## Reference List

1 Bishop MH, Shoemaker WC, Appel PL, Meade P, Ordog GJ, Wasserberger J, et al. *Prospective, randomized trial of survivor values of cardiac index, oxygen delivery, and oxygen consumption as resuscitation endpoints in severe trauma.* J Trauma 1995 May; 38(5): 780-7.

2 Boyd O, Grounds RM, Bennett ED. *A randomized clinical trial of the effect of deliberate peri-operative increase of oxygen delivery on mortality in high-risk surgical patients.* JAMA 1993 Dec 8; 270(22): 2699-707.

3 Wilson J, Woods I, Fawcett J, Whall R, Dibb W, Morris C, et al. *Reducing the risk of major elective surgery: randomised controlled trial of preoperative optimisation of oxygen delivery.* BMJ 1999 Apr 24; 318 (7191): 1099-103.

4 Tuchschmidt J, Fried J, Astiz M, Rackow E. *Elevation of cardiac output and oxygen delivery improves outcome in septic shock.* Chest 1992 Jul; 102(1): 216-20.

5 Hayes MA, Timmins AC, Yau EH, Palazzo M, Hinds CJ, Watson D. *Elevation of systemic oxygen delivery in the treatment of critically ill patients.* N Engl J Med 1994 Jun 16; 330(24): 1717-22.

6 Gattinoni L, Brazzi L, Pelosi P, Latini R, Tognoni G, Pesenti A, et al. *A trial of goal-oriented hemodynamic therapy in critically ill patients.* SvO2 Collaborative Group. N Engl J Med 1995 Oct 19; 333(16): 1025-32.

7 Rivers E, Nguyen B, Havstad S, Ressler J, Muzzin A, Knoblich B, et al. *Early goal-directed therapy in the treatment of severe sepsis and septic shock.* N Engl J Med 2001 Nov 8; 345(19): 1368-77.

8 Singer M, De S, V, Vitale D, Jeffcoate W. *Multiorgan failure is an adaptive, endocrine-mediated, metabolic response to overwhelming systemic inflammation.* Lancet 2004 Aug 7; 364(9433): 545-8.

# Peri-operative volume management guided by venous or tissue oxygenation

# Niels H. Secher

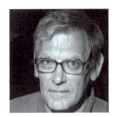

**Current position**
Anaesthesiologist
Copenhagen University Hospital
Denmark

Head of the Human Cardiovascular Research Laboratory, associated to the Copenhagen Muscle Research Centre.

Prof Secher has published more than 300 articles within human cardiovascular control summarised into the concept of "normovolaemia" and its importance for maintained regional perfusion including cerebral blood flow during surgery.

# Peri-operative volume management guided by venous or tissue oxygenation

Niels H. Secher

*Department of Anaesthesia*
*Rigshospitalet 2041*
*University of Copenhagen, Denmark*

Intravenous administration of fluid and blood is a common in-hospital procedure because a volume deficit of only little more than 500 ml leads to hypovolaemic shock. Yet, too much fluid leads to peripheral or pulmonary oedema and delayed surgical healing and accurate peri-operative fluid management is difficult because there is no agreed goal to guide the treatment.

*a volume deficit of only little more than 500 ml leads to hypovolaemic shock*

Here it is emphasised that in supine healthy humans, preload to the heart is large enough to secure cardiac output[2]. Accordingly, the supine surgical patient has a volume deficit when cardiac output is limited by preload to the heart. Conversely, administration of blood can be continued until the volume load does not result in any further increase in cardiac output or stroke volume, i.e. *normovolaemia* is established.

For the administration of whole blood and with no change in haematocrit, such provision of volume ensures that the patient has the central blood volume that he normally has when lying down. On the other hand, peri-operative fluid administration is most often with isotonic saline or Ringer-lactate followed by a plasma expander. For the surgical patient, administration of red cells is reserved for situations where the adult patient has a bleed of more than approximately one litre.

With planned haemodilution for the peri-operative patient, it is considered that there is a reverse relationship between cardiac output and haematocrit[4]. The anaemic patient has a remarkably large cardiac output, while cardiac output is low for the hypoxic pulmonary patient with a high haematocrit.

*The anaemic patient has a remarkably large cardiac output*

## Venous oxygenation

When an increase in cardiac output or stroke volume is used for goal-directed volume therapy, the patient receives a larger volume load than the one he would have during supine rest because of the increase in flow by haemodilution. Conversely, an increasing cardiac output with decreasing haematocrit means that mixed or central venous oxygen saturation stays statistically unchanged over a range of isovolaemic haemodilution[4]. Accordingly, goal-directed volume therapy becomes independent of the chosen preparation for the volume load when it is directed to provide the patient with maximal venous oxygen saturation rather than with a maximal cardiac output or stroke volume[7]. A strategy for volume management based on venous oxygen saturation requires that a central venous line or a pulmonary artery catheter is in place and it is convenient if both catheters can report a continuous value. Volume management can then be directed to maintain the normal average venous oxygen saturation of 75% for supine humans[2]. For the anaesthetised or intensive patient, however, venous oxygen saturation may be both lower (72%)[3] and higher (85%)[1]. Besides the vasodilatation induced by the anaesthetics and regional anaesthesia, vasodilatation may be provoked by fever, sepsis or by the disease itself as exemplified by liver insufficiency. Thus during experimental heating of healthy subjects to a core temperature of 38° C, venous oxygen saturation may increase to 97% and the subject becomes ill when venous oxygen saturation is reduced to 85% because the central blood volume is attenuated. Representative values for different types of surgical patients are not available, but for goal-directed therapy, the individual maximal venous oxygen saturation is identified with a reported range of 56% to 92%[6]. The expected response can be guided in that a volume deficit of ~ 100 ml corresponds to a 1% decrease in venous oxygen saturation for the adult patient.

*A strategy for volume management based on venous oxygen saturation*

## Tissue oxygenation

Hypovolaemia is associated with vasoconstriction to skeletal muscles and muscle oxygenation decreases[5]. Muscle oxygenation may be monitored by near-infrared spectroscopy (NIRS) and for the ambulatory patient, unlikely to be provided with a central venous catheter, non-invasive recording of muscle oxygenation is an acceptable alternative to venous oxygenation for managing volume therapy.

Equally, NIRS is used to monitor cerebral oxygenation non-invasively[5]. While venous or muscle oxygenation provide values suited for managing of fluid therapy, the recording of brain oxygenation may be taken to represent a quality control of the treatment, i.e. that the volume management is able to maintain cerebral oxygenation during surgery.

*non-invasive recording of muscle oxygenation is an acceptable alternative to venous oxygenation*

Continuous evaluation of cerebral oxygenation is important especially for procedures involving hypotensive anaesthesia. Under such procedures blood pressure is lower than the pressure considered to represent the lower limit of cerebral autoregulation. Yet, the NIRS determined cerebral oxygenation, and hence blood flow, may be preserved to a mean arterial pressure of 37 mmHg. For the individual patient, however, the lower limit of cerebral autoregulation may be higher, e.g. 55 mmHg and, if hypotension is caused by a reduction in central blood volume, the lower limit of cerebral autoregulation increases towards 80 mmHg, or to a level similar to the pressure that normal people possess. Without the recording of brain (often forehead) oxygenation, it remains unknown whether a low blood pressure is acceptable for maintained brain function.

## Conclusion

Of these different strategies for goal-directed volume management during the peri-operative period, only an evaluation based on establishing a maximal cardiac output or stroke volume has been validated for clinical outcome with the oesophageal Doppler as the dominant method. However, there is no reason to believe that other methods for continuous detection of cardiac output or stroke volume of the heart should provide the patients with a markedly different volume load.

*only an evaluation based on establishing a maximal cardiac output or stroke volume has been validated for clinical outcome with the oesophageal Doppler*

As indicated, a strategy for goal-directed volume therapy based on administration of crystalloids and/or plasma expanders provides the patient, at least in principle, with a larger load than a strategy based on venous or tissue oxygenation. As the volume load reached during maximising stroke volume is outcome validated, it is suggested that the peri-operative patient is provided with a volume that is approximately 500 ml larger than the one that elicits a maximal venous or muscle oxygenation. It is also suggested that the quality not only of volume management but also of anaesthesia is taken into consideration when assessing the ability of the procedure to maintain cerebral oxygenation.

# Reference List

1 Ejlersen E, Skak C, Møller K, Pott F, Secher N. *Central cardiovascular variables at a maximal mixed venous saturation in severe hepatic failure.* Transplant Proc 1995; 27: 3506-3507.

2 Harms MP, Van Lieshout JJ, Jenstrup M, Pott F, Secher NH. *Postural effects on cardiac output and mixed venous oxygen saturation in humans.* Exp Physiol 2003; 88: 611-616.

3 Jenstrup M, Ejlersen E, Mogensen T, Secher NH. *A maximal central venous oxygen saturation (SvO2max) for the surgical patient.* Acta Anaesthesiol Scand 1995; 39 (Suppl 107): 29-32.

4 Krantz T, Warberg J, Secher NH. *Venous oxygen saturation during norvolaemic haemodilution in the pig.* Acta Anaesthesiol Scand 2005; 49: 1149-1156.

5 Madsen PL, Secher NH. *Near-infrared oximetry of the brain.* Prog Neurobiol 1999; 58: 541-560.

6 Madsen PL, Skak C, Rasmussen A, Secher NH. *Interference of cerebral near-infrared oximetry in patients with icterus.* Anesth Analg 2000; 90: 489-493.

7 Secher NH, Van Lieshout JJ. *Normovolaemia defined by central blood volume and venous oxygen saturation.* Clin Exp Pharm Physiol 2005; 32: 901-910.

# Peri-operative renal failure
– a great fluid perspective

# Tony Roche

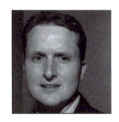

**Current position**
Assistant Professor
Department of Anesthesiology
Duke University Medical Center
Durham, NC, USA

Director
Department of Anesthesiology Liver Transplant
Hepatobiliary Fellowship Program
Duke University Medical Center, USA

Honorary Fellow
University College London, UK

# Peri-operative renal failure – a great fluid perspective
Tony Roche

*Department of Anesthesiology
Duke University Medical Center
Durham, NC, USA*

Acute renal failure (ARF) is a devastating peri-operative complication, characterised by a decline in glomerular filtration, and a rapid rise in nitrogenous waste products (e.g. urea and creatinine). It is observed in 15-30% of critically ill patients[1,2], carrying a mortality rate of 15-72%, depending on patient population, number of organ system failure, comorbidities, and cause of ARF[3,4]. It is commonly defined as an acute rise of approximately 45 mcmol/L over a baseline creatinine below 200 mcmol/L, or a twofold increase over baseline creatinine concentration. More recently, the RIFLE criteria have been developed by a multidisciplinary consensus panel to classify the extent of renal failure[5]. These criteria are based on degree of elevation of creatinine from baseline, as well as urine output[5].

*More recently, the RIFLE criteria have been developed*

Risk factors associated with ARF are age, hypovolaemia, hypotension, sepsis, pre-existing renal, hepatic or cardiac dysfunction, diabetes mellitus, nephrotoxins, immunosuppressive agents, non-steroidal anti-inflammatory drugs, intravenous contrast media, and multiple organ dysfunction syndrome[2]. Furthermore, ischaemia-reperfusion, aortic clamping, embolic phenomena, inflammatory response to surgery, and pigments (e.g. myoglobins) play an important peri-operative role.

Measurement of renal function can be performed in a number of ways. Changes in peri-operative serum creatinine concentration has been used as a marker, however, little consensus exists regarding exact limits to define varying levels of impairment or failure. Twenty-four hour creatinine clearance remains the gold standard. A two-hour creatinine clearance has been advocated in critical care settings, as it appears to correlate well with the 24 hour clearance[6]. As seen with the RIFLE criteria, serum creatinine change and urine output can also be employed as markers of renal function. On the other hand, peri-operative urine output has been notoriously poor at predicting post-operative renal impairment or failure[7]. This may be for a number of reasons, possibly that the majority of these studies are underpowered to detect clinically significant differences in renal function between study groups.

> *peri-operative urine output ...notoriously poor at predicting post-operative renal impairment*

Further serum and urine markers of renal function have been described recently, e.g. Cystatin C, and NGAL. Cystatin C, a cysteine proteinase inhibitor which is produced by all nucleated cells, is a good indicator of glomerular filtration as it accumulates in renal failure[8]. NGAL (neutrophil gelatinase-associated lipocalcin) is a protein expressed by ischaemic renal tubular cells, which, if present in the urine of peri-operative patients, has been shown to predict acute renal failure[9]. Besides these markers, proteinuria is also indicative of renal dysfunction.

Although hypovolaemia and dehydration are associated with ARF, there are scant data implicating their roles peri-operatively. Schroeder et al performed a retrospective analysis of a low central venous pressure (CVP), or fluid restrictive technique versus a normal fluid management technique in 151 patients undergoing liver transplantation surgery[10]. They found a significantly higher incidence of post-operative ARF, higher peak serum creatinine levels, lower intra-operative urine output, and increased 30-day mortality in the low-CVP group, despite these patients having lower pre-operative severity of disease indices. Although these data are compelling, it needs to be remembered that the study is retrospective from two centers; one center uses low-CVP, while the other employs a normal CVP technique.

Despite the benefit of peri-operative optimization, or goal-directed therapy (GDT) to the gastrointestinal system, days in ICU, and hospital length of stay, there are no distinct proven benefits to the renal system. Certain studies have shown improved urine output associated with GDT, but no differences have been observed in rates of renal impairment or failure[11-14].

*Despite the benefit of peri-operative optimization... there are no distinct proven benefits to the renal system*

The fluid restriction literature describes peri-operative weight gain as a measure of fluid therapy, or volume of fluid administered. This body of work suggests restricting the amount of peri-operative fluid administered to a predefined maximum limit. In a study of 172 surgical patients, Brandstrup et al investigated a restricted (peri-operative weight gain limited to 1 kg) versus a standard peri-operative fluid regimen on patient outcomes[15]. Interestingly, there was no difference in renal outcomes, suggesting that the restrictive group may in fact have received appropriate fluid management (and not necessarily "restrictive"), and that such therapy does not lead to an increased risk of renal failure.

This leads to the perennial question of crystalloids versus colloids. Firstly, not all crystalloids are the same. Balanced salt preparations appear to cause greater urine output when compared with 0.9% Sodium Chloride (NaCl) preparations[16], a process which is likely to be due to NaCl-associated hyperchloraemia causing renal vasoconstriction[17]. It should be remembered that these data have not translated to differences in peri-operative ARF rates. In a study of patients undergoing coronary angiography, the choice of 0.9% NaCl IV fluid therapy significantly reduced contrast nephropathy when compared with a technique using 0.45% NaCl with dextrose solution[18]. Another study investigating a sodium bicarbonate and dextrose solution versus a 0.9% NaCl solution found that the bicarbonate-based fluid regime significantly reduced contrast nephropathy[19]. No such studies as these last two have been performed in peri-operative patients.

*NaCl-associated hyperchloraemia causing renal vasoconstriction*

The second question of IV fluids returns to the crystalloid-colloid debate. In the single biggest randomized controlled study of IV fluid therapy in critically ill patients, the SAFE study examined 0.9% NaCl versus 4% albumin solution (suspended in 0.9% NaCl). No difference was observed between the type of fluid used and any renal outcomes[20].

The third question regarding type of fluid revolves around the colloids particularly. A study by Schortgen et al investigated 129 critically ill patients with severe sepsis, randomized to receive a 6% hydroxyethyl starch (HES, 200 kDa, 0.6 substitution ratio) or a 3% modified fluid gelatin solution for IV volume expansion[21]. They observed an increased rate of ARF in the HES group, together with greater oliguria rates, and greater peak creatinine concentrations. This is consistent with previous reports of renal impairment associated with HES IV fluids. On the other hand, Boldt et al recently published an investigation of 50 patients undergoing major abdominal surgery, randomized to receive either 5% albumin solution or a third generation 6% HES (130 kDa, 0.4 substitution ratio), both with Lactated Ringer's solution for crystalloid therapy[22]. In their study, they found no difference in renal failure, or in any urine markers of renal tubular integrity.

*hypovolaemia and severe dehydration remain significant concerns*

In summary, it appears that despite the lack of adequate peri-operative data, hypovolaemia and severe dehydration remain significant concerns for peri-operative ARF. Well-designed fluid "restrictive" regimens are not associated with adverse renal outcomes, however this should not be confused with peri-operative patients being subjected to receiving little to no IV fluids at all. Besides differences observed in urine output (itself a poor marker of peri-operative renal function), no data exist to suggest saline based or balanced electrolyte IV fluids are associated with improved renal outcomes. Albumin and gelatin solutions are not currently associated with adverse renal outcomes, however there remains a degree of concern with HES IV fluids and patients with pre-existing, or at risk of, renal impairment. This may not be the same with all HES compounds, also depending on the protocol for adjunctive crystalloid administration.

With the significant lack of peri-operative studies, one is destined to learn lessons from other fields, such as those of contrast nephropathy, severe sepsis, as well as other critical care medicine. Administering no fluid is bad, too much fluid can be bad – the peri-operative challenge is getting it right!

*Administering no fluid is bad, too much fluid can be bad – the peri-operative challenge is getting it right!*

## Reference List

1 Hou SH, Bushinsky DA, Wish JB et al. *Hospital-acquired renal insufficiency: a prospective study.* Am J Med 1983; 74: 243-8.

2 Brivet FG, Kleinknecht DJ, Loirat P, Landais PJ. *Acute renal failure in intensive care units, causes, outcome, and prognostic factors of hospital mortality; a prospective, multicenter study. French Study Group on Acute Renal Failure.* Crit Care Med 1996; 24: 192-8.

3 Liano F, Junco E, Pascual J et al. *The spectrum of acute renal failure in the intensive care unit compared with that seen in other settings. The Madrid Acute Renal Failure Study Group.* Kidney Int Suppl 1998; 66: S16-24.

4 Metnitz PG, Krenn CG, Steltzer H et al. *Effect of acute renal failure requiring renal replacement therapy on outcome in critically ill patients.* Crit Care Med 2002; 30: 2051-8.

5 Bellomo R, Ronco C, Kellum JA et al. *Acute renal failure – definition, outcome measures, animal models, fluid therapy and information technology needs: the Second International Consensus Conference of the Acute Dialysis Quality Initiative (ADQI) Group.* Crit Care 2004; 8: R204-12.

6 Sladen RN, Endo E, Harrison T. *Two-hour versus 22-hour creatinine clearance in critically ill patients.* Anesthesiology 1987; 67: 1013-6.

7 Alpert RA, Roizen MF, Hamilton WK et al. *Intraoperative urinary output does not predict postoperative renal function in patients undergoing abdominal aortic revascularization.* Surgery 1984; 95: 707-11.

8 Levin A, Cystatin C. *Serum creatinine, and estimates of kidney function: searching for better measures of kidney function and cardiovascular risk.* Ann Intern Med 2005; 142: 586-8.

9 Mishra J, Dent C, Tarabishi R et al. *Neutrophil gelatinase-associated lipocalin (NGAL) as a biomarker for acute renal injury after cardiac surgery.* Lancet 2005; 365: 1231-8.

10 Schroeder RA, Collins BH, Tuttle-Newhall E et al. *Intraoperative fluid management during orthotopic liver transplantation.* J Cardiothorac Vasc Anesth 2004; 18: 438-41.

11 Gan TJ, Soppitt A, Maroof M et al. *Goal-directed intraoperative fluid administration reduces length of hospital stay after major surgery.* Anesthesiology 2002; 97: 820-6.

12 Mythen MG, Webb AR. *Peri-operative plasma volume expansion reduces the incidence of gut mucosal hypoperfusion during cardiac surgery.* Arch Surg 1995; 130: 423-9.

13 Wakeling HG, McFall MR, Jenkins CS et al. *Intraoperative oesophageal Doppler guided fluid management shortens postoperative hospital stay after major bowel surgery.* Br J Anaesth 2005; 95: 634-42.

14 Wilson J, Woods I, Fawcett J et al. *Reducing the risk of major elective surgery: randomised controlled trial of preoperative optimisation of oxygen delivery.* BMJ 1999; 318: 1099-103.

15 Brandstrup B, Tonnesen H, Beier-Holgersen R et al. *Effects of intravenous fluid restriction on postoperative complications: comparison of two peri-operative fluid regimens: a randomized assessor-blinded multicenter trial.* Ann Surg 2003; 238: 641-8.

16 Williams EL, Hildebrand KL, McCormick SA, Bedel MJ. The effect of intravenous lactated Ringer's solution versus 0.9% sodium chloride solution on serum osmolality in human volunteers. Anesth Analg 1999; 88: 999-1003.

17 Wilcox CS. *Regulation of renal blood flow by plasma chloride.* J Clin Invest 1983; 71: 726-35.

18 Mueller C, Buerkle G, Buettner HJ et al. *Prevention of contrast media-associated nephropathy: randomized comparison of 2 hydration regimens in 1620 patients undergoing coronary angioplasty.* Arch Intern Med 2002; 162: 329-36.

19 Merten GJ, Burgess WP, Gray LV et al. *Prevention of contrast-induced*

*nephropathy with sodium bicarbonate: a randomized controlled trial.* Jama 2004; 291: 2328-34.

20 Finfer S, Bellomo R, Boyce N et al. *A comparison of albumin and saline for fluid resuscitation in the intensive care unit.* N Engl J Med 2004; 350: 2247-56.

21 Schortgen F, Lacherade JC, Bruneel F et al. *Effects of hydroxyethyl-starch and gelatin on renal function in severe sepsis: a multicentre randomised study.* Lancet 2001; 357: 911-6.

22 Boldt J, Scholhorn T, Mayer J et al. *The value of an albumin-based intravascular volume replacement strategy in elderly patients undergoing major abdominal surgery.* Anesth Analg 2006; 103: 191-9.

# Peri-operative fluid management – bowel function/oral nutrition, fast-tracking and design issues

# Henrik Kehlet

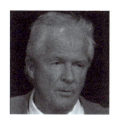

### Current position

Professor Henrik Kehlet is a gastrointestinal surgeon and former Professor of Surgery, Copenhagen University and is now Professor of Peri-operative Therapy, Head of Section of Surgical Pathophysiology, The Juliane Marie Centre, Rigshospitalet, Copenhagen University.

Prof Kehlet has published more than 600 articles within peri-operative pathophysiology, pain relief and surgical outcome summarized into the concept of "fast-track surgery", which also includes a focus on peri-operative fluid management.

# Peri-operative fluid management – bowel function/oral nutrition, fast-tracking and design issues
Henrik Kehlet

*Section of Surgical Pathophysiology*
*The Juliane Marie Centre*
*Rigshospitalet, Copenhagen*

Post-operative outcome is determined by multiple factors[1] where peri-operative fluid management may influence several organ functions and thereby recovery. PONV and paralytic ileus are important determinants of recovery in some types of surgery and nausea and vomiting has been reduced in about 30% of minor procedures (i.e. < 24 hours post-op stay)[2-4] when administering > 1 litre intraoperatively compared with less. In major procedures avoidance of fluid excess or goal-directed therapy has reduced ileus in 4 of 8 randomised studies[5-12] which is clinically relevant since it allows for early oral nutrition which elsewhere has been demonstrated to improve outcome[13].

*there is no doubt that peri-operative fluid management may influence recovery*

Although there is no doubt that peri-operative fluid management may influence recovery, the available studies do not allow final conclusions regarding key issues on timing, composition and exact amount of fluids, use of vasopressors, specific problems with central neuroaxial blockade. Furthermore, there is a need for more procedure-specific data, since post-operative fluid kinetics may be procedure-dependent. However, most importantly, all randomised trials except two[3,12] have design problems in that peri-operative care principles have not been described in detail and revised according to available evidence, and several studies have included different types of procedures, hindering exact interpretation. Future fluid-outcome studies should be randomised, with well-defined evidence-based components of care (fast-track surgery[1]) and initially with a focus on functional outcomes:

> *all randomised trials except two have design problems*

- pulmonary: conventional tests and SpO2;

- cardiac: orthostatic function, balance, exercise tolerance, ischaemia, SV, CO, tissue 02;

- PONV, ileus, nutrition, wound function: tissue 02/infection;

- endocrine responses: vasoactive hormones;

- inflammatory responses: CRP, IL-6, coagulation/fibrinolysis and achievement of well-defined evidence-based discharge criteria, all in well-defined, procedure-specific studies[14].

## Reference List

1 Kehlet H, Dahl JB. *Anaesthesia, surgery, and challenges in postoperative recovery.* Lancet 2003; 362(9399): 1921-8.

2 Holte K, Kehlet H. *Compensatory fluid administration for preoperative dehydration – does it improve outcome?* Acta Anaesthesiol Scand 2002; 46: 1089-93.

3 Holte K, Klarskov B, Christensen DS, Lund C, Nielsen KG, Bie P, Kehlet H. *Liberal versus restrictive fluid administration to improve recovery after laparoscopic cholecystectomy: a randomized, double-blind study.* Ann Surg 2004; 240: 892-9.

4 Maharaj CH, Kallam SR, Malik A, Hassett P, Grady D, Laffey JG. *Preoperative intravenous fluid therapy decreases postoperative nausea and pain in high risk patients.* Anesth & Analg 2005; 100: 675-82.

5 Nisanevich V, Felsenstein I, Almogy G, Weissman C, Einav S, Matot I. *Effect of intraoperative fluid management on outcome after intra-abdominal surgery.* Anesthesiology 2005; 103: 25-32.

6 Kabon B, Akca O, Taguchi A, Nagele A, Jebadurai R, Arkilic CF, Sharma N, Ahluwalia A, Galandiuk S, Fleshman J, Sessler DI, Kurz A. *Supplemental intravenous crystalloid administration does not reduce the risk of surgical wound infection.* Anesth Analg 2005; 101(5): 1546-53.

7 Kassel et al. J R Soc Med 1996; 89: 249-252.

8 Lobo DN, Bostock KA, Neal KR, Perkins AC, Rowlands BJ, Allison SP. *Effect of salt and water balance on recovery of gastrointestinal function after elective colonic resection: a randomised controlled trial.* Lancet 2002; 359: 1812-1818.

9 Conway DH, Mayall R, Abdul-Latif MS, Gilligan S, Tackaberry C. *Randomised controlled trial investigating the influence of intravenous fluid titration using oesophageal Doppler monitoring during bowel surgery.* Anaesthesia 2002; 57: 845-849.

10 Gan TJ, Soppitt A, Maroof M et al. *Goal directed intraoperative fluid administration reduces length of hospital stay after major surgery.* Anesthesiology 2002; 97: 820-6.

11 Wakeling HG, McFall MR, Jenkins CS et al. *Intraoperative oesophageal Doppler guided fluid management shortens postoperative hospital stay after major bowel surgery.* Br J Anaesth 2005; 95: 634-642.

12 Holte et al. 2006 (submitted).

13 Lewis SJ, Egger M, Sylvester PA, Thomas S. *Early enteral feeding versus "nil by mouth" after gastrointestinal surgery: systematic review and meta-analysis of controlled trials.* BMJ 2001; 323 (7316): 773-6.

14 Holte K, Kehlet H. *Fluid therapy and surgical outcome in elective surgery – a need for reassessment in fast-track surgery – A systematic review.* J Am Coll Surg 2006; 202: 971-989.

Restricted fluid regimen and volumes of colloid/crystalloid

# Birgitte Brandstrup

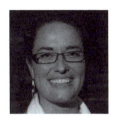

### Current position
Birgitte Brandstrup M.D. in 1992
and Ph.D in 2003, both from
The University of Copenhagen

### Publications
Ph.D thesis, articles, letters, a book
and book chapters on the subject
'Peri-operative fluid management'
in general and, in particular,
'Restricted intravenous fluid therapy'

# Restricted fluid regimen and volumes of colloid/crystalloid
Birgitte Brandstrup

*Surgical Gastroenterological Department*
*Bispebjerg University Hospital*
*Copenhagen, Denmark*

*Background:* Peri-operative fluid management is the subject of much controversy, and the results of the clinical trials investigating the effect of fluid therapy on outcome of surgery seem contradictory.

*Aim:* To review the evidence behind current standard fluid therapy, and thereby analyse if the so-called "restricted fluid regimen" (see the below) in fact is "restricted" or merely designed to avoid fluid overload.

*Results:* Current standard fluid therapy is not at all evidence based:

*1. Glucose containing fluid is a good choice for the basal requirements.*
The fluid lost by perspiration and during preoperative fasting is primarily water, but replacement with water (i.e. oral fluid or i.v. Glucose 5%) has previously been discouraged because of concerns about aspiration and enhancement of the rise in plasma glucose caused by the surgical stress. Clinical trials have, however, shown that

preoperative glucose administration either intravenously or orally reduce the post-operative cellular insulin resistance[1], increase well-being[2], and improve post-operative muscle strength[3].

*2. The evaporative loss from the abdominal wound is very small.*
It depends on the size of the incision and the exposure of the intestines and ranges from 2.1 g/h (small incisions with slightly exposed viscera) to 32.2 g/h (major incisions with completely exteriorised viscera)[4].

*3. The non-anatomical third space loss most probably does not exist.*
It is believed that the surgical trauma *per se* causes a *contraction of the ECV*, with a volume of extra cellular fluid sequestered in a compartment where it is unavailable for measurement with a tracer or for the regeneration of lost plasma. This phenomenon was first described in 1960 in a trial of dogs subjected to haemorrhagic shock[5]: compared to the ECV before bleeding, the ECV measured during shock was much smaller than anticipated from the volume of lost blood. The same observation was made in patients undergoing abdominal surgery: despite correction for external losses, the measured ECV during surgery was found largely diminished (up to 3.7 litres) compared to similar measurements before surgery[6]. A systematic review of the literature concerning measurements of

*All other studies...have not been able to find a contraction of the ECV*

ECV-changes in surgery and haemorrhagic shock reveals, however, that only trials utilizing the $SO^{35}$-tracer and very short equilibration time (20-30 minutes) have demonstrated this non-anatomical third space loss. All other studies identified, utilizing various different tracers, multiple sampling techniques, and longer equilibration times, have not been able to find a contraction of the ECV either during surgery or during haemorrhagic shock. Furthermore, investigators utilizing the labelled bromide tracer have found the opposite of a third space loss: corrected for the lost blood, an expansion of the ECV rather than a contraction was found following surgery[7].

*4. The fluid volume accumulated in traumatised tissue (the anatomical third space loss) during elective surgery is very small.*

Before, during, or after surgery the disease and/or the surgical trauma may cause fluid to accumulate in a transcellular – or the interstitial space. The volume of fluid accumulated in the interstitial space of traumatized tissue is highly influenced by the administration of intravenous crystalloids. In a study of rabbits it was found that the formation of a small bowel anastomosis caused a 5-10% increase in the water content of the surrounding tissue if no fluid was administered. The oedema doubled when 15 ml/kg/h of Hartman's solution was given[8]. If equivalent changes occur in humans, 2.5-5 ml may accumulate around a large bowel anastomosis if no crystalloid is administered, and 5-10 ml may accumulate if 15 ml/kg/h is given. A volume of this magnitude is of no importance for the development of hypovolemia, but may be important for the healing of the anastomosis.

## 5. *Extra fluid for preloading of neuroaxial blockade is not effective but may cause post-operative fluid overload.*

Early studies suggested preloading to reduce the incidence of hypotension in 20-35% of patients, but this has not been confirmed in clinical randomised trials of preloading versus no preloading[9,10]. Neither the decrease in blood pressure nor the need for pressure substances was significantly altered by the fluid preloading of the neuroaxial blockade.

*[not] significantly altered by the fluid preloading of the neuroaxial blockade*

## 6. *Outcome trials*

The trials of "goal-directed fluid therapy" giving extra HES to maximal stroke volume have shown contradictory results. The difference in results may have many causes, but one of the most important may be a lax attitude towards "standard fluid therapy" ending up testing various "standard fluid regimens" versus "even more fluid". Another important issue may be the lack of control or registration of pre-and post-operative intravenous fluid therapy.

The principles of "restricted intravenous fluid therapy" have only been tested in abdominal surgery, but the results have been a consistent improvement of outcome[11-13]. The trials of different fluid volumes administered during outpatient surgery confirm that replacement of fluid lost improves outcome.

## Conclusion

"Restricted intravenous fluid therapy" is not "restricted", but avoids fluid overload by replacing only the fluid actually lost during surgery.

- Preoperative fasting longer than 2 hours should be avoided. Water loss should be replaced with a water preparation (unless contraindications for i.v. glucose exist).

- The non-anatomical third space loss does not exist or the volume is very small.

- The evaporative losses and the anatomical third space loss need only be considered during extended surgery (and are replaced by medicinal water).

- Oedema can be minimised by a volume for volume replacement of lost blood with a colloid. Because of the delayed measuring of the blood loss an extra volume of maximum of 500 ml HES is permitted.

- Early enteral feeding and drinking is commenced post-operatively.

## Reference List

1 Nygren J, Soop M, Thorell A, Sree Nair K, Ljungqvist O. *Preoperative oral carbohydrates and postoperative insulin resistance.* Clin Nutr 1999; 18: 117-120.

2 Hausel J, Nygren J, Almström C, et al. *Peri-operative oral carbohydrate improve well being after elective colorectal surgery.* Clin Nutr 1999; 18 suppl 1: 21.

3 Henriksen MG. *Effects of preoperative oral carbohydrates and peptides on postoperative endocrine response, mobilization, nutrition and muscle function in abdominal surgery.* Acta Anesthesiol Scand 2003; 47: 191-199.

4 Lamke LO, Nilsson GE, Reithner HL. Water loss by evaporation from the abdominal cavity during surgery. Acta Chir Scand 1977; 143: 279-84.

5 Shires T, Brown FT, Canizaro PC, Summerville N. *Distributional changes in extra cellular fluid during acute hemorrhagic shock.* Surg Forum 1960; 11: 115-117.

6 Shires T, Williams J, Brown F. *Acute changes in extracellular fluids associated with major surgical procedures.* Ann Surg 1961; 154: 803-810.

7 Brandstrup B, Svendsen C, Engquist A. *Haemorrhage and operation cause a contraction of the extra cellular space needing replacement – Evidence and implications? A systematic review.* Surgery 2006; 139: 419-432.

8 Chan STF, Kapadia CR, Johnson AW, Radcliff AG, Dudley HAF. *Extracellular fluid volume expansion and third space sequestration at the site of small bowel anastomosis.* Br J Surg 1983; 70: 36-39.

9 Kinsella SM, Pirlet M, Mills MS, Tuckey JP, Thomas TA. *Randomised study of intravenous fluid preload before epidural analgesia during labour.* Br J Anaesth 2000; 85: 311-313.

10 Kubli M, Shennan AH, Seed PT, O'Sullivan G. *A randomised controlled trial of fluid pre-loading before low dose epidural analgesia for labour.* Int J Obstet Anesth 2003; 12: 256-260.

11 Brandstrup B, Tønnesen H, Beier-Holgersen R, Hjortsø E, Ørding H, Lindorff-Larsen K, Rasmussen MS, Lanng C, Wallin L, and The Danish Study Group on Peri-operative Fluid therapy. *Effects of intravenous fluid restriction on postoperative complications: comparison of two peri-operative fluid regimens. A randomised assessor blinded multi centre trial.* Ann Surg 2003; 238: 641-648.

12 Lobo DN, Bostock KA, Neal KR, Perkins AC, Rowlands BJ, Allison SP. *Effect of salt and water balance on recovery of gastrointestinal function after elective colonic resection: a randomised controlled trial.* Lancet 2002; 359: 1812-1818.

13 Nisanevich V, Felsenstein I, Almogy G, Weissman C, Einav S, Matot I. *Effect of intraoperative fluid management on outcome after intraabdominal surgery.* Anesthesiology 2005; 103: 25-32.

# Fluid therapy and coagulation

# Mike James

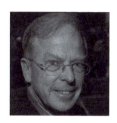

### Current position
Professor and Head of
Department of Anaesthesia
University of Cape Town
South Africa

### Special interests
Magnesium as a cardiovascular drug, fluid therapy, anaesthesia for endocrine surgery, anaesthesia for vascular surgery and the management of hypertension in anaesthesia including pre-eclampsia

Sports fanatic

# Fluid therapy and coagulation
Mike James

*Department of Anaesthesia*
*University of Cape Town*
*Observatory 7925*
*Cape Town, South Africa*

## Crystalloids

Crystalloids are generally assumed to have no intrinsic effect on coagulation, other than dilutional effects. However, 50 years ago Tocantins and colleagues demonstrated that dilution of blood with any of the solutions that they tested accelerated coagulation[1]. Eight years later, Monkhouse showed that two-and threefold dilutions of plasma with saline increased production of thrombin, and speculated that this may be due to an induced imbalance between thrombin and antithrombin[2]. In a clinical study of acute normovolaemic haemodilution, using a mixture of 50% albumin and 50% Ringer's lactate, the r- and k-times on the TEG were shortened following haemodilution and the non-activated partial thromboplastin time was also reduced[3].

*dilution of blood with any of the solutions that they tested accelerated coagulation*

An *in vitro* study of volunteer blood showed that 20% dilution with saline or a gelatin (Haemaccel®) resulted in accelerated clot formation as measured by the TEG compared to undiluted control blood samples. Haemodilution with saline also increased final clot strength (MA), whereas haemodilution with gelatin decreased MA[4]. Subsequent studies with temperature control and balanced, buffered crystalloid solutions with pH 7.4 showed similar effects[5]. *In vivo* haemodilution with 1L of either 0.9% saline or HES 200/0.5 (Haes-Steril®) in conscious volunteers showed comparable results for saline but, HES was virtually without effect on coagulation[6]. In this study, there were marked reductions in both fibrinogen and antithrombin III (ATIII) of approximately double the magnitude of the haemodilution. This was evidence of enhanced coagulation with consumption of both fibrinogen and ATIII[6]. This suggested that an imbalance between procoagulant and anticoagulant factors was a likely explanation for the observations. Dose-response studies using saline dilutions ranging from 10% to 60% showed that haemodilution of up to 40% resulted in enhanced coagulation, with the peak effect occurring between 30 and 40%. A study of haemodilution in which calcium was controlled, suggested that >60% haemodilution with calcium-containing fluids was necessary before impairment of coagulation by crystalloid haemodilution could be observed[7].

*an imbalance between procoagulant and anticoagulant factors*

Clinical studies have reported similar effects. Two studies[8,9] reported progressive increases in the coagulability that correlated with the volume of crystalloid resuscitation fluids administered during surgical procedures. Martin and colleagues showed that Ringer's lactate induced a hypercoagulable state in surgical patients that persisted well into the post-operative period, but was not seen when the resuscitation solution containing hydroxyethyl starch in a balanced salt solution was administered[10]. The conclusions regarding crystalloid haemodilution seem clear. Crystalloid solutions enhance coagulation up to 40% dilution. Further haemodilution with crystalloids will not significantly impair the rate of clot formation until haemodilution is > 60%, provided the levels of ionized calcium are maintained within the normal range, although clot strength will diminish slightly, presumably due to platelet dilution. The possibility that this enhanced coagulation may be beneficial during resuscitation of a bleeding patient may partly explain other observations that crystalloid resuscitation appears to be associated with a better outcome in trauma than colloid resuscitation[11]. On the other hand, the potential adverse effects of excessive coagulation including deep vein thrombosis remain possible, but currently unproven, risks of crystalloid fluid therapy. The possibility that excessive coagulation induced by crystalloids may predispose to disseminated intravascular coagulation is also worthy of consideration. There are currently insufficient data upon which to base firm conclusions in this area.

### Colloids

Theoretically, if haemodilution creates an imbalance between procoagulant and anticoagulant factors, then colloid solutions ought to exert a similar procoagulant effect to that seen with crystalloids. There is some evidence that this may be the case, but the influence of various colloids on the coagulation process itself offsets the effects of dilution of anticoagulant factors. The individual colloid solutions appear to be quite different in this regard, although the general belief is that the dextrans exert the greatest effects on inhibition of coagulation, followed by the starches, with the gelatins and albumin having the least inhibitory effect. However, there are considerable differences between the different types of starch solutions and these need to be considered individually.

## Dextrans

The dextrans are branched chain polysaccharides with average molecular weights in the range of 40-70 kilo Daltons (kD). The dextrans exert significant effects on coagulation and can markedly impair coagulation[12]. Beneficial effects have also been claimed for the dextrans in minimising DVT risks and maintaining the patency of vascular grafts[13] and they have been shown to diminish the incidence of cerebral micro-embolic phenomena following carotid endarterectomy[14]. This effect seems to be greatest with the hyperoncotic 10% dextran 40 compared to the isotonic 6% dextran 60/70. However, in moderate doses, there is little evidence that the use of the dextrans results in increased surgical bleeding[15]. Dextrans cause

> *The dextrans exert significant effects on coagulation and can markedly impair coagulation*

reductions in the effective levels of the von Willebrand factor (vWF) and the associated factor VIII (vWF/VIII), accelerate the activation of protein C by factor Xa[16], and diminish clot strength[17]. Patients with underlying coagulation disorders, particularly von Willebrand's disease or haemophilia, should not receive these products and they should be used with great care in patients receiving anticoagulant therapy, including low molecular weight heparins.

### Gelatins

The gelatins are polydisperse molecules, but with a smaller average molecular weight than the other synthetic colloids, in the range of 30-35 kD. There are two types of gelatin: the polygelines in which polypeptides are linked through a urea bridge (Haemaccel®), and the succinylated (fluid) gelatins (Gelofusin®, Gelofundin®). These differ in both their average MW and electrical charge, as well as in their propensity to produce allergic reactions. Several comparative studies have suggested that the gelatins have a lesser effect on coagulation than other colloids[18,19,20,21] and some studies have suggested an acceleration of coagulation by gelatin with moderate haemodilution, both *in vitro*[4] and *in vivo*[22], albeit with decreased MA. Consequently, the gelatins are widely regarded as having minimal effects on coagulation, and for this reason there is no 24-hour dosage limit imposed on these intravenous solutions. This is not a universally accepted view, and there are several

*there are several studies suggesting impaired clot strength* studies suggesting impaired clot strength[23,4] and a decreased rate of clot formation particularly at dilutions in excess of 40%[24,25,26]. Gelofusine® may have a greater anticoagulant effect than does Haemaccel®, possibly due to the greater negative charge on the molecule in the former preparation, but not due to the differences in calcium content[27]. As with dextran, impairment of coagulation by the gelatins appears to be mediated through a reduction in the activity of vWF and decreased platelet aggregation[28]. The clinical relevance of the influence of gelatins on coagulation is not established, and only 2 studies suggested an increase in surgical bleeding associated with their use[28,29]. It seems reasonable to conclude that the older gelatins have less effect on coagulation than most of the other colloid preparations. The possibility that gelatins (particularly the succinylated variety) may impair coagulability should be borne in mind, especially in patients receiving anticoagulants or who may have other causes of impaired blood clotting[30].

*The clinical relevance of the influence of gelatins on coagulation is not established*

## Hydroxyethyl starch

Starch preparations have differing pharmacological properties depending on the extent of molar substitution (MS) and the position of the substitution on the molecule. The pharmacological effects depend primarily on the molecular weight of the starch particles within the plasma. This *in vivo* MW is the result of the initial MW and of the rate of breakdown of the starch in plasma which depends primarily on the MS and C2/C6 ratio, with the highly substituted HES (MS > 0.5) being relatively poorly metabolized[31]. The effects of HES on haemostasis has recently been reviewed[32].

High MW MS HES (MW > 400 kD, MS > 0.6, the only form available in the US) have significant adverse effects on coagulation, particularly if the daily dosage limit of 20 ml/kg is exceeded although increased consumption of blood and platelets was observed after cardiac surgery with as little as 10 ml/kg of high MW starch[33,34]. The main mechanism of action of HES appears to be through a combination of the large starch molecules with the vWF/VIII complex. High MS HES (480/0.7) decreased factor VIII by 50% after infusion of 1L[35]. The MS appears to be more important than the initial MW[36]. Prolonged infusions (over 10 days) of HES 200/0.62 (*in vivo* MW 120 kD) resulted in marked impairment of the activated partial thromboplastin time and reductions in the vWF/VIII complex below the critical value of 30%, whereas HES 200/0.5 (*in vivo* MW 84 kD), had no effect beyond that of haemodilution[37]. Interestingly, it has been suggested that patients with blood group O were more likely to show reduced vWF activity after the use of HES 200/0.6 than patients with other blood groups[38]. High *in vivo* MW HES can also bind to platelets leading to increased platelet degradation[31]. A study investigating the effects of HES on the expression of activated glycoprotein IIb/IIIa complex using flow

*High MW MS HES have significant adverse effects on coagulation*

cytometry showed that HES 450/0.7-0.8, HES 200/0.6-0.66, and HES 70/0.5-0.55 prolonged closure times and reduced glycoprotein IIb/IIIa expression, whereas saline and HES 130/0.4 had no significant effect on platelet variables[39]. Modification of the high MW HES by changing the suspending solution from saline to a balanced salt solution may partially offset some of the adverse effects of the HES[40,41], and there is some evidence of reduced blood loss with this preparation in a clinical setting[42]. Clinical studies on HES 130/0.4 (*in vivo* MW 70 kD) have suggested that it has minimal effect on coagulation measures and on clinical blood loss[43,44,45,46].

*Clinical studies on HES 130/0.4 have suggested that it has minimal effect on coagulation*

## Albumin

Albumin is assumed to be without coagulation effects. In a laboratory study, profound impairment of coagulation as measured by the TEG was found using albumin at 50% haemodilution, whereas HES had only moderate effects and saline maintained coagulation[47]. However, this study did not control for calcium concentrations in the diluted samples, and we have found that calcium binding by albumin profoundly decreases ionized calcium in a laboratory setting[48]. A recent study found that succinylated gelatin and HES 200/0.5 impaired coagulation after cardiac surgery, but albumin did not[29]. It seems reasonable, therefore, to conclude that albumin probably exerts some minor effects on coagulation, the nature of which is not yet established.

In conclusion, haemodilution with crystalloids enhances coagulation by a mechanism that probably involves differential dilutions of anticoagulant factors. This may be beneficial in the resuscitation of a bleeding patient but may be harmful if it leads to be exaggerated coagulation in the post-operative period. The gelatins generally interfere with coagulation to a relatively small degree, whereas the dextrans exert significant impairment on coagulation. The effects on coagulation of HES depend on the *in vivo* MW of the starch product, with the high MW, high MS starches causing significant inhibition of coagulation, while the newer, medium MW, low MS starch products have almost no adverse effects on coagulation.

## Reference List

1 Tocantins LM, Carroll RT, Holburn RH. *The clot accelerating effect of dilution on blood and plasma. Relation to the mechanism of coagulation of normal and hemophiliac blood.* Blood 1951; 6: 720-739.

2 Monkhouse FC. *Relationship between antithrombin and thrombin levels in plasma and serum.* American Journal of Physiology 1959; 197: 984-988.

3 Bergmann H, Blauhut B, Brucke P, Necek S, Vinazzer H. *[Early influence of acute preoperative haemodilution with human albumin and Ringer's lactate on coagulation (author's transl)].* Anaesthesist 1976; 25: 175-180.

4 Ruttmann TG, James MF, Viljoen JF. *Haemodilution induces a hypercoagulable state.* Br J Anaesth 1996; 76: 412-414.

5 Ruttmann TG, James MF, Wells KF. *Effect of 20% in vitro haemodilution with warmed buffered salt solution and cerebrospinal fluid on coagulation.* Br J Anaesth 1999; 82: 110-111.

6 Ruttmann TG, James MF, Aronson I. *In vivo investigation into the effects of haemodilution with hydroxyethyl starch (200/0.5) and normal saline on coagulation.* Br J Anaesth 1998; 80: 612-616.

7 Roche AM, James MF, Grocott MP, Mythen MG. *Coagulation effects of in vitro serial haemodilution with a balanced electrolyte hetastarch solution compared with a saline-based hetastarch solution and lactated Ringer's solution.* Anaesthesia 2002; 57: 950-957.

8 Tuman KJ, Spiess BD, McCarthy RJ, Ivankovich AD. *Effects of progressive blood loss on coagulation as measured by thrombelastography.* Anesth Analg 1987; 66: 856-863.

9 Ng KF, Lo JW. *The development of hypercoagulability state, as measured by thrombelastography, associated with intraoperative surgical blood loss.* Anaesth Intensive Care 1996; 24: 20-25.

10 Martin G, Bennett-Guerrero E, Wakeling H et al. *A prospective,*

*randomized comparison of thromboelastographic coagulation profile in patients receiving lactated Ringer's solution, 6% hetastarch in a balanced-saline vehicle, or 6% hetastarch in saline during major surgery.* J Cardiothorac Vasc Anesth 2002; 16: 441-446.

11 Choi PT, Yip G, Quinonez LG, Cook DJ. *Crystalloids vs. colloids in fluid resuscitation: a systematic review.* Crit Care Med 1999; 27: 200-210.

12 Blanloeil Y, Trossaert M, Rigal JC, Rozec B. *[Effects of plasma substitutes on hemostasis].* Ann Fr Anesth Reanim 2002; 21: 648-667.

13 Bergman A, Andreen M, Blomback M. *Plasma substitution with 3% dextran-60 in orthopaedic surgery: influence on plasma colloid osmotic pressure, coagulation parameters, immunoglobulins and other plasma constituents.* Acta Anaesthesiol Scand 1990; 34: 21-29.

14 Lennard N, Smith J, Dumville J et al. *Prevention of postoperative thrombotic stroke after carotid endarterectomy: the role of transcranial Doppler ultrasound.* J Vasc Surg 1997; 26: 579-584.

15 Bergman A, Andreen M, Blomback M. *Plasma substitution with 3% dextran-60 in orthopaedic surgery: influence on plasma colloid osmotic pressure, coagulation parameters, immunoglobulins and other plasma constituents.* Acta Anaesthesiol Scand 1990; 34: 21-29.

16 Rezaie AR. *Rapid activation of protein C by factor Xa and thrombin in the presence of polyanionic compounds.* Blood 1998; 91: 4572-4580.

17 Levy G, Mak CC, Nhean H. *[Hemodilution in vitro and parameters of hemostasis].* Ann Anesthesiol Fr 1979; 20: 784-788.

18 Konrad C, Markl T, Schuepfer G, Gerber H, Tschopp M. *The effects of in vitro hemodilution with gelatin, hydroxyethyl starch, and lactated Ringer's solution on markers of coagulation: an analysis using SONOCLOT.* Anesth Analg 1999; 88: 483-488.

19 Mortier E, Ongenae M, De Baerdemaeker L et al. *In vitro evaluation of the effect of profound haemodilution with hydroxyethyl starch 6%, modified fluid gelatin 4% and dextran 40 10% on coagulation profile measured by thromboelastography.* Anaesthesia 1997; 52: 1061-1064.

20 Petroianu GA, Liu J, Maleck WH, Mattinger C, Bergler WF. *The effect of in vitro hemodilution with gelatin, dextran, hydroxyethyl starch, or Ringer's solution on Thrombelastograph.* Anesth Analg 2000; 90: 795-800.

21 Mortelmans YJ, Vermaut G, Verbruggen AM et al. *Effects of 6% hydroxyethyl starch and 3% modified fluid gelatin on intravascular volume and coagulation during intraoperative hemodilution.* Anesth Analg 1995; 81: 1235-1242.

22 Karoutsos S, Nathan N, Lahrimi A, Grouille D, Feiss P, Cox DJ. *Thrombelastogram reveals hypercoagulability after administration of gelatin solution.* Br J Anaesth 1999; 82: 175-177.

23 Mardel SN, Saunders FM, Allen H et al. *Reduced quality of clot formation with gelatin-based plasma substitutes.* Br J Anaesth 1998; 80: 204-207.

24 Brazil EV, Coats TJ. *Sonoclot coagulation analysis of in-vitro haemodilution with resuscitation solutions.* J R Soc Med 2000; 93: 507-510.

25 de Jonge E, Levi M, Berends F, van der Ende AE, ten Cate JW, Stoutenbeek CP. *Impaired haemostasis by intravenous administration of a gelatin-based plasma expander in human subjects.* Thromb Haemost 1998; 79: 286-290.

26 Egli GA, Zollinger A, Seifert B, Popovic D, Pasch T, Spahn DR. *Effect of progressive haemodilution with hydroxyethyl starch, gelatin and albumin on blood coagulation.* Br J Anaesth 1997; 78: 684-689.

27 Coats TJ, Heron M. *Does calcium cause the different effects of Gelofusine and Haemaccel on coagulation?* Emerg Med J 2006; 23: 193-194.

28 Tabuchi N, de Haan J, Gallandat Huet RC, Boonstra PW, van Oeveren W. *Gelatin use impairs platelet adhesion during cardiac surgery.* Thromb Haemost 1995; 74: 1447-1451.

29 Niemi TT, Suojaranta-Ylinen RT, Kukkonen SI, Kuitunen AH. *Gelatin and hydroxyethyl starch, but not albumin, impair hemostasis after cardiac surgery.* Anesth Analg 2006; 102: 998-1006.

30 de Jonge E, Levi M. *Effects of different plasma substitutes on blood coagulation: a comparative review.* Crit Care Med 2001; 29: 1261-1267.

31 Treib J, Haass A, Pindur G, Treib W, Wenzel E, Schimrigk K. *Influence of intravascular molecular weight of hydroxyethyl starch on platelets.* Eur J Haematol 1996; 56: 168-172.

32 Kozek-Langenecker SA. *Effects of hydroxyethyl starch solutions on hemostasis.* Anesthesiology 2005; 103: 654-660.

33 Brutocao D, Bratton SL, Thomas JR, Schrader PF, Coles PG, Lynn AM. *Comparison of hetastarch with albumin for postoperative volume expansion in children after cardiopulmonary bypass.* J Cardiothorac Vasc Anesth 1996; 10: 348-351.

34 Cope JT, Banks D, Mauney MC et al. *Intraoperative hetastarch infusion impairs hemostasis after cardiac operations.* Ann Thorac Surg 1997; 63: 78-82.

35 Stump DC, Strauss RG, Henriksen RA, Petersen RE, Saunders R. *Effects of hydroxyethyl starch on blood coagulation, particularly factor VIII.* Transfusion 1985; 25: 349-354.

36 von Roten I, Madjdpour C, Frascarolo P et al. *Molar substitution and C2/C6 ratio of hydroxyethyl starch: influence on blood coagulation.* Br J Anaesth 2006; 96: 455-463.

37 Treib J, Haass A, Pindur G et al. *Increased haemorrhagic risk after repeated infusion of highly substituted medium molecular weight hydroxyethyl starch.* Arzneimittelforschung 1997; 47: 18-22.

38 Huraux C, Ankri AA, Eyraud D et al. *Hemostatic changes in patients receiving hydroxyethyl starch: the influence of ABO blood group.* Anesth Analg 2001; 92: 1396-1401.

39 Franz A, Braunlich P, Gamsjager T, Felfernig M, Gustorff B, Langenecker SA. *The effects of hydroxyethyl starches of varying molecular weights on platelet function.* Anesth Analg 2001; 92: 1402-1407.

40 Roche AM, James MF, Grocott MP, Mythen MG. *Coagulation effects of in vitro serial haemodilution with a balanced electrolyte hetastarch*

*solution compared with a saline-based hetastarch solution and lactated Ringer's solution.* Anaesthesia 2002; 57: 950-955.

41 Roche AM, James MF, Bennett-Guerrero E, Mythen MG. *A head-to-head comparison of the in vitro coagulation effects of saline-based and balanced electrolyte crystalloid and colloid intravenous fluids.* Anesth Analg 2006; 102: 1274-1279.

42 Gan TJ, Bennett-Guerrero E, Phillips-Bute B et al. *Hextend, a physiologically balanced plasma expander for large volume use in major surgery: a randomized phase III clinical trial. Hextend Study Group.* Anesth Analg 1999; 88: 992-998.

43 Langeron O, Doelberg M, Ang ET, Bonnet F, Capdevila X, Coriat P. *Voluven, a lower substituted novel hydroxyethyl starch (HES 130/0.4), causes fewer effects on coagulation in major orthopedic surgery than HES 200/0.5.* Anesth Analg 2001; 92: 855-862.

44 Vogt NH, Bothner U, Lerch G, Lindner KH, Georgieff M. *Large-dose administration of 6% hydroxyethyl starch 200/0.5 total hip arthroplasty: plasma homeostasis, hemostasis, and renal function compared to use of 5% human albumin.* Anesth Analg 1996; 83: 262-268.

45 Gallandat Huet RC, Siemons AW, Baus D et al. *A novel hydroxyethyl starch (Voluven) for effective perioperative plasma volume substitution in cardiac surgery.* Can J Anaesth 2000; 47: 1207-1215.

46 Van der Linden PJ, De Hert SG, Deraedt D et al. *Hydroxyethyl starch 130/0.4 versus modified fluid gelatin for volume expansion in cardiac surgery patients: the effects on perioperative bleeding and transfusion needs.* Anesth Analg 2005; 101: 629-34, table.

47 Tobias MD, Wambold D, Pilla MA, Greer F. *Differential effects of serial hemodilution with hydroxyethyl starch, albumin, and 0.9% saline on whole blood coagulation.* J Clin Anesth 1998; 10: 366-371.

48 Roche AM, James MF, Bennett-Guerrero E, Mythen MG. A head-to-head comparison of the in vitro coagulation effects of saline-based and balanced electrolyte crystalloid and colloid intravenous fluids. Anesth Analg 2006; 102: 1274-1279.

# Interviews

Interviews with specialists

# Interviews

**On the disk** available with this book Prof Monty Mythen interviews the following specialists.

These interviews can also be viewed at www.rockfacemedicine.com

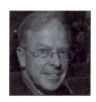

❝The older estimates of third space loss are almost certainly excessive but we don't know by how much❞

Mike James

**Fluid therapy and coagulation**

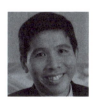

❝Combining monitoring with a clear management algorithm... will improve patient outcomes❞

T J Gan

**Goal-directed fluid administration – peri-operative perspectives**

"There is no doubt that peri-operative fluid management may influence recovery"

### Henrik Kehlet

**Peri-operative fluid management – bowel function/oral nutrition, fast-tracking and design issues**

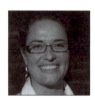

"Restricted intravenous fluid therapy is not restricted but avoids fluid overload by replacing only the fluid actually lost during surgery"

### Birgitte Brandstrup

**Restricted fluid regimen and volumes of colloid/crystalloid**

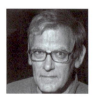

"A volume deficit of only little more than 500ml leads to hypovolaemic shock"

### Niels H. Secher

**Peri-operative volume management guided by venous or tissue oxygenation**

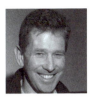

## "'Goal-directed therapy' reduces mortality and improves outcomes"

### Mike Grocott

**Goal-directed fluid administration – ICU perspectives**

# Bibliography

# Bibliography

The following pages contain an alphabetical list of references. This list can also be found on the disk that is available with this book. By selecting the **More Information** option on the disk followed by the **Bibliography** option you can access a pdf file with live links to the relevant abstracts. This pdf file is also available at www.rockfacemedicine.com.

Ali SZ, Taguchi A, Holtmann B, Kurz A. *Effect of supplemental preoperative fluid on postoperative nausea and vomiting.* Anaesthesia 2003; 58: 780-4.

Alpert RA, Roizen MF, Hamilton WK et al. *Intraoperative urinary output does not predict postoperative renal function in patients undergoing abdominal aortic revascularization.* Surgery 1984; 95: 707-11.

Bellomo R, Ronco C, Kellum JA et al. *Acute renal failure - definition, outcome measures, animal models, fluid therapy and information technology needs: the Second International Consensus Conference of the Acute Dialysis Quality Initiative (ADQI) Group.* Crit Care 2004; 8: R204-12.

Bender JS, Smith-Meek MA, Jones CE. *Routine pulmonary artery catheterization does not reduce morbidity and mortality of elective vascular surgery: results of a prospective, randomized trial.* Annals of Surgery 1997; 226: 229-36; discussion 36-7.

Bergman A, Andreen M, Blomback M. *Plasma substitution with 3% dextran-60 in orthopaedic surgery: influence on plasma colloid osmotic pressure, coagulation parameters, immunoglobulins and other plasma constituents.* Acta Anaesthesiol Scand 1990; 34: 21-29.

Bergmann H, Blauhut B, Brucke P, Necek S, Vinazzer H. *[Early influence of acute preoperative haemodilution with human albumin and ringer's lactate on coagulation (author's transl)].* Anaesthesist 1976; 25: 175-180.

Berlauk JF, Abrams JH, Gilmour IJ et al. *Preoperative optimization of cardiovascular hemodynamics improves outcome in peripheral vascular surgery. A prospective, randomized clinical trial [see comments].* Annals of Surgery 1991; 214: 289-97; discussion 98-9.

Bishop MH, Shoemaker WC, Appel PL, Meade P, Ordog GJ, Wasserberger J, et al. *Prospective, randomized trial of survivor values of cardiac index, oxygen delivery, and oxygen consumption as resuscitation endpoints in severe trauma.* J Trauma 1995 May; 38(5): 780-7.

Blanloeil Y, Trossaert M, Rigal JC, Rozec B. *[Effects of plasma substitutes on hemostasis].* Ann Fr Anesth Reanim 2002; 21: 648-667.

Boldt J, Scholhorn T, Mayer J et al. *The value of an albumin-based intravascular volume replacement strategy in elderly patients undergoing major abdominal surgery.* Anesth Analg 2006; 103: 191-9.

Boldt J. *Fluid management of patients undergoing abdominal surgery – more questions than answers?* Eur J Anaesthesiol. 2006; 23: 631-40.

Boyd O, Grounds RM, Bennett ED. *A randomized clinical trial of the effect of deliberate peri-operative increase of oxygen delivery on mortality in high-risk surgical patients.* JAMA 1993 Dec 8; 270(22): 2699-707.

Boyd O, Tremblay RE, Spencer FC, and Bahnson HT. *Estimation of Cardiac Output Soon After Cardiac Surgery With Cardiopulmonary Bypass.* Annals of Surgery 1959; 150: 613-25. Abstract not available.

Brandstrup B, Svendsen C, Engquist A. *Haemorrhage and operation cause a contraction of the extra cellular space needing replacement - Evidence and implications? A systematic review.* Surgery 2006; 139: 419-432.

Brandstrup B, Tønnesen H, Beier-Holgersen R, Hjortsø E, Ørding H, Lindorff-Larsen K, Rasmussen MS, Lanng C, Wallin L, and The Danish Study Group on Perioperative Fluid therapy. *Effects of intravenous fluid restriction on postoperative complications: comparison of two perioperative fluid regimens. A randomised assessor blinded multi centre trial.* Ann Surg 2003; 238: 641-648.

Brazil EV, Coats TJ. *Sonoclot coagulation analysis of in-vitro haemodilution with resuscitation solutions.* J R Soc Med 2000; 93: 507-510.

Brivet FG, Kleinknecht DJ, Loirat P, Landais PJ. *Acute renal failure in intensive care units-causes, outcome, and prognostic factors of hospital mortality; a prospective, multicenter study. French Study Group on Acute Renal Failure.* Crit Care Med 1996; 24: 192-8.

Brutocao D, Bratton SL, Thomas JR, Schrader PF, Coles PG, Lynn AM. *Comparison of hetastarch with albumin for postoperative volume expansion in children after cardiopulmonary bypass.* J Cardiothorac Vasc Anesth 1996; 10: 348-351.

Chan ST, Kapadia CR, Johnson AW, Radcliff AG, Dudley HAF. *Extracellular fluid volume expansion and third space sequestration at the site of small bowel anastomosis.* Br J Surg 1983; 70: 36-39.

Choi PT, Yip G, Quinonez LG, Cook DJ. *Crystalloids vs. colloids in fluid resuscitation: a systematic review.* Crit Care Med 1999; 27: 200-210.

Clowes GaDG, LRM. *Circulatory Response to Trauma of Surgical Patients.* Metabolism 1960; 9: 67-81. Abstract not available

Coats TJ, Heron M. *Does calcium cause the different effects of Gelofusine and Haemaccel on coagulation?* Emerg Med J 2006; 23: 193-194.

Conway DH, Mayall R, Abdul-Latif MS, Gilligan S, Tackaberry C. *Randomised controlled trial investigating the influence of intravenous fluid titration using oesophageal Doppler monitoring during bowel surgery.* Anaesthesia 2002; 57: 845-849.

Cope JT, Banks D, Mauney MC et al. *Intraoperative hetastarch infusion impairs hemostasis after cardiac operations.* Ann Thorac Surg 1997; 63: 78-82.

Critchley LA, Conway F. *Hypotension during subarachnoid anaesthesia: haemodynamic effects of colloid and metaraminol [see comments].* British Journal of Anaesthesia 1996; 76: 734-6.

de Jonge E, Levi M, Berends F, van der Ende AE, ten Cate JW, Stoutenbeek CP. *Impaired haemostasis by intravenous administration of a gelatin-based plasma expander in human subjects.* Thromb Haemost 1998; 79: 286-290.

de Jonge E, Levi M. *Effects of different plasma substitutes on blood coagulation: a comparative review.* Crit Care Med 2001; 29: 1261-1267.

Egli GA, Zollinger A, Seifert B, Popovic D, Pasch T, Spahn DR. *Effect of progressive haemodilution with hydroxyethyl starch, gelatin and albumin on blood coagulation.* Br J Anaesth 1997; 78: 684-689.

Ejlersen E, Skak C, Møller K, Pott F, and Secher N. *Central cardiovascular variables at a maximal mixed venous saturation in severe hepatic failure.*

Transplant Proc 27: 3506-3507, 1995. Abstract not available.

Ewaldsson CA, Hahn RG. *Kinetics and extravascular retention of acetated ringer's solution during isoflurane or propofol anesthesia for thyroid surgery.* Anesthesiology 2005; 103: 460-9.

Finfer S, Bellomo R, Boyce N et al. *A comparison of albumin and saline for fluid resuscitation in the intensive care unit.* N Engl J Med 2004; 350: 2247-56.

Fleming A, Bishop M, Shoemaker W et al. *Prospective trial of supranormal values as goals of resuscitation in severe trauma.* Archives of Surgery 1992; 127: 1175-9; discussion 9-81.

Franz A, Braunlich P, Gamsjager T, Felfernig M, Gustorff B, Kozec-Langenecker SA. *The effects of hydroxyethyl starches of varying molecular weights on platelet function.* Anesth Analg 2001; 92: 1402-1407.

Gallandat Huet RC, Siemons AW, Baus D et al. *A novel hydroxyethyl starch (Voluven) for effective perioperative plasma volume substitution in cardiac surgery.* Can J Anaesth 2000; 47: 1207-1215.

Gan TJ, Bennett-Guerrero E, Phillips-Bute B et al. *Hextend, a physiologically balanced plasma expander for large volume use in major surgery: a randomized phase III clinical trial. Hextend Study Group.* Anesth Analg 1999; 88: 992-998.

Gan TJ, Soppitt A, Maroof M et al. *Goal-directed intraoperative fluid administration reduces length of hospital stay after major surgery.* Anesthesiology 2002; 97: 820-6.

Gattinoni L, Brazzi L, Pelosi P, Latini R, Tognoni G, Pesenti A, et al. *A trial of goal-oriented hemodynamic therapy in critically ill patients. SvO2 Collaborative Group.* N Engl J Med 1995 Oct 19; 333(16): 1025-32.

Grocott MP, Mythen MG, Gan TJ: *Peri-operative fluid management and clinical outcomes in adults.* Anesth Analg 2005; 100: 1093-106.

Hahn RG, Drobin D, Stahle L: *Volume kinetics of Ringer's solution in female volunteers.* Br J Anaesth. 1997; 78: 144-8.

Harms MP, Van Lieshout JJ, Jenstrup M, Pott F, and Secher NH. *Postural effects on cardiac output and mixed venous oxygen saturation in humans.* Exp Physiol 88: 611-616, 2003.

Hausel J, Nygren J, Almström C, et al. *Perioperative oral carbohydrate improve well being after elective colorectal surgery.* Clin Nutr 1999; 18 suppl 1:21. Abstract not available.

Hayes MA, Timmins AC, Yau EH, Palazzo M, Hinds CJ, Watson D. *Elevation of systemic oxygen delivery in the treatment of critically ill patients.* N Engl J Med 1994 Jun 16; 330(24): 1717-22.

Henriksen MG et al. *Effects of preoperative oral carbohydrates and peptides on post-operative endocrine response, mobilization, nutrition and muscle function in abdominal surgery.* Acta Anesthesiol Scand 2003; 47: 191-199.

Holte K, Foss NB, Andersen J, Lund C, Valentiner L, Bie P, Kehlet H. *Liberal vs restrictive fluid management in fast-track colonic surgery. A randomized, double-blind study. (submitted).* Abstract not available.

Holte K, Foss NB, Svensen C, Lund C, Madsen JL, Kehlet H. *Epidural anesthesia, hypotension, and changes in intravascular volume.* Anesthesiology 2004; 100: 281-6.

Holte K, Hahn RG, Ravn L, Bertelsen KG, Hansen S, Kehlet H. *The influence of liberal vs restrictive intra-operative fluid management on the elimination of a postoperative intravenous fluid load (submitted).* Abstract not available.

Holte K, Kehlet H. *Compensatory fluid administration for preoperative dehydration – does it improve outcome?* Acta Anaesthesiol Scand 2002; 46: 1089-93.

Holte K, Kehlet H. *Fluid therapy and surgical outcome in elective surgery – a need for reassessment in fast-track surgery – A systematic review.* J Am Coll Surg 2006; 202: 971-989. Abstract not available.

Holte K, Klarskov B, Christensen DS, Lund C, Nielsen KG, Bie P, Kehlet H. *Liberal versus restrictive fluid administration to improve recovery after laparoscopic cholecystectomy: a randomized, double-blind study.* Ann Surg 2004; 240: 892-9.

Holte K, Kristensen BB, Valentiner L, Foss NB, Husted H, Kehlet H. *Liberal vs restrictive fluid management in knee arthroplasty. A randomized, double-blind study (submitted).* Abstract not available.

Holte K, Sharrock NE, Kehlet H. *Pathophysiology and clinical implications of peri-operative fluid excess.* Br J Anaesth 2002; 89: 622-32. Abstract not available.

Hou SH, Bushinsky DA, Wish JB et al. *Hospital-acquired renal insufficiency: a prospective study.* Am J Med 1983; 74: 243-8.

Huraux C, Ankri AA, Eyraud D et al. *Hemostatic changes in patients receiving hydroxyethyl starch: the influence of ABO blood group.* Anesth Analg 2001; 92: 1396-1401.

Jenstrup M, E Ejlersen, T Mogensen, and NH Secher. *A maximal central venous oxygen saturation (SvO2max) for the surgical patient.* Acta Anaesthesiol Scand 1995; 39 (Suppl 107): 29-32.

Kabon B, Akca O, Taguchi A, Nagele A, Jebadurai R, Arkilic CF, Sharma N, Ahluwalia A, Galandiuk S, Fleshman J, Sessler DI, Kurz A. *Supplemental intravenous crystalloid administration does not reduce the risk of surgical wound infection.* Anesth Analg 2005; 101(5): 1546-53.

Karoutsos S, Nathan N, Lahrimi A, Grouille D, Feiss P, Cox DJ. *Thrombelastogram reveals hypercoagulability after administration of gelatin solution.* Br J Anaesth 1999; 82: 175-177.

Kehlet H, Dahl JB. *Anaesthesia, surgery, and challenges in postoperative recovery.* Lancet. 2003; 362(9399): 1921-8.

Kinsella SM, Pirlet M, Mills MS, Tuckey JP, Thomas TA. *Randomised study of intravenous fluid preload before epidural analgesia during labour.* Br J Anaesth 2000; 85: 311-313.

Konrad C, Markl T, Schuepfer G, Gerber H, Tschopp M. *The effects of in vitro hemodilution with gelatin, hydroxyethyl starch, and lactated Ringer's solution on markers of coagulation: an analysis using SONOCLOT.* Anesth Analg 1999; 88: 483-488.

Kozek-Langenecker SA. *Effects of hydroxyethyl starch solutions on hemostasis.* Anesthesiology 2005; 103: 654-660. Abstract not available.

Krantz T, Warberg J, and Secher NH. *Venous oxygen saturation during norvolaemic haemodilution in the pig.* Acta Anaesthesiol Scand 2005; 49: 1149-1156.

Kubli M, Shennan AH, Seed PT, O'Sullivan G. *A randomised controlled trial of fluid pre-loading before low dose epidural analgesia for labour.* Int J Obstet Anesth 2003; 12: 256-260.

Lamke LO, Nilsson GE, Reithner HL. *Water loss by evaporation from the abdominal cavity during surgery.* Acta Chir Scand 1977; 143: 279-84.

Langeron O, Doelberg M, Ang ET, Bonnet F, Capdevila X, Coriat P. *Voluven, a lower substituted novel hydroxyethyl starch (HES 130/0.4), causes fewer effects on coagulation in major orthopedic surgery than HES 200/0.5.* Anesth Analg 2001; 92: 855-862.

Lennard N, Smith J, Dumville J et al. *Prevention of post-operative thrombotic stroke after carotid endarterectomy: the role of transcranial Doppler ultrasound.* J Vasc Surg 1997; 26: 579-584.

Levin A, Cystatin C. *Serum creatinine, and estimates of kidney function: searching for better measures of kidney function and cardiovascular risk.* Ann Intern Med 2005;142: 586-8. Abstract not available.

Levy G, Mak CC, Nhean H. *[Hemodilution in vitro and parameters of hemostasis].* Ann Anesthesiol Fr 1979; 20: 784-788. Abstract not available.

Lewis SJ, Egger M, Sylvester PA, Thomas S. *Early enteral feeding versus "nil by mouth" after gastrointestinal surgery: systematic review and meta-analysis of controlled trials.* BMJ 2001; 323 (7316): 773-6.

Liano F, Junco E, Pascual J et al. *The spectrum of acute renal failure in the intensive care unit compared with that seen in other settings. The Madrid Acute Renal Failure Study Group.* Kidney Int Suppl 1998; 66: S16-24.

Lobo DN, Bostock KA, Neal KR, Perkins AC, Rowlands BJ, Allison SP. *Effect of salt and water balance on recovery of gastrointestinal function after elective colonic resection: a randomised controlled trial.* Lancet 2002; 359: 1812-1818.

Madsen PL and Secher NH. *Near-infrared oximetry of the brain.* Prog Neurobiol 1999; 58: 541-560.

Madsen PL, Skak C, Rasmussen A, and Secher NH. *Interference of cerebral near-infrared oximetry in patients with icterus.* Anesth Analg 2000; 90: 489-493.

Maharaj CH, Kallam SR, Malik A, Hassett P, Grady D, Laffey JG: *Preoperative intravenous fluid therapy decreases post-operative nausea and pain in high risk patients.* Anesthesia & Analgesia 2005; 100: 675-82.

Mardel SN, Saunders FM, Allen H et al. *Reduced quality of clot formation with gelatin-based plasma substitutes.* Br J Anaesth 1998; 80: 204-207.

Martin G, Bennett-Guerrero E, Wakeling H et al. *A prospective, randomized comparison of thromboelastographic coagulation profile in patients receiving lactated Ringer's solution, 6% hetastarch in a balanced-saline vehicle, or 6% hetastarch in saline during major surgery.* J Cardiothorac Vasc Anesth 2002; 16: 441-446.

Merten GJ, Burgess WP, Gray LV et al. *Prevention of contrast-induced nephropathy with sodium bicarbonate: a randomized controlled trial.* Jama 2004; 291: 2328-34.

Metnitz PG, Krenn CG, Steltzer H et al. *Effect of acute renal failure requiring renal replacement therapy on outcome in critically ill patients.* Crit Care Med 2002; 30: 2051-8.

Mishra J, Dent C, Tarabishi R et al. *Neutrophil gelatinase-associated lipocalin (NGAL) as a biomarker for acute renal injury after cardiac surgery.* Lancet 2005; 365: 1231-8.

Monkhouse FC. *Relationship between antithrombin and thrombin levels in plasma and serum.* American Journal of Physiology 1959; 197: 984-988.

Mortelmans YJ, Vermaut G, Verbruggen AM et al. *Effects of 6% hydroxyethyl starch and 3% modified fluid gelatin on intravascular volume and coagulation during intraoperative hemodilution.* Anesth Analg 1995; 81: 1235-1242.

Mortier E, Ongenae M, De Baerdemaeker L et al. *In vitro evaluation of the effect of profound haemodilution with hydroxyethyl starch 6%, modified fluid gelatin 4% and dextran 40 10% on coagulation profile measured by thromboelastography.* Anaesthesia 1997; 52: 1061-1064.

Mueller C, Buerkle G, Buettner HJ et al. *Prevention of contrast media-associated nephropathy: randomized comparison of 2 hydration regimens in 1620 patients undergoing coronary angioplasty.* Arch Intern Med 2002; 162: 329-36.

Mythen MG, Webb AR. *Perioperative plasma volume expansion reduces the incidence of gut mucosal hypoperfusion during cardiac surgery.* Archives of Surgery 1995; 130: 423-9.

Ng KF, Lo JW. *The development of hypercoagulability state, as measured by thrombelastography, associated with intraoperative surgical blood loss.* Anaesth Intensive Care 1996; 24: 20-25.

Niemi TT, Suojaranta-Ylinen RT, Kukkonen SI, Kuitunen AH. *Gelatin and hydroxyethyl starch, but not albumin, impair hemostasis after cardiac surgery.* Anesth Analg 2006; 102: 998-1006.

Nisanevich V, Felsenstein I, Almogy G, Weissman C, Einav S, Matot I. *Effect of intraoperative fluid management on outcome after intraabdominal surgery.* Anesthesiology 2005; 103: 25-32.

Nygren J, Soop M, Thorell A, Sree Nair K, Ljungqvist O. *Preoperative oral carbohydrates and postoperative insulin resistance.* Clin Nutr 1999; 18: 117-120.

Olsson J, Svensen CH, Hahn RG: *The volume kinetics of acetated Ringer's solution during laparoscopic cholecystectomy.* Anesthesia & Analgesia 2004; 99: 1854-60.

Petroianu GA, Liu J, Maleck WH, Mattinger C, Bergler WF. *The effect of in vitro hemodilution with gelatin, dextran, hydroxyethyl starch, or Ringer's solution on Thrombelastograph.* Anesth Analg 2000; 90: 795-800.

Polonen P, Ruokonen E, Hippelainen M et al. *A prospective, randomized study of goal-oriented hemodynamic therapy in cardiac surgical patients.* Anesth Analg 2000; 90: 1052-9.

Rezaie AR. *Rapid activation of protein C by factor Xa and thrombin in the presence of polyanionic compounds.* Blood 1998; 91: 4572-4580.

Rivers E, Nguyen B, Havstad S, Ressler J, Muzzin A, Knoblich B, et al. *Early goal-directed therapy in the treatment of severe sepsis and septic shock.* N Engl J Med 2001 Nov 8; 345(19): 1368-77.

Roche AM, James MF, Bennett-Guerrero E, Mythen MG. *A head-to-head comparison of the in vitro coagulation effects of saline-based and balanced electrolyte crystalloid and colloid intravenous fluids.* Anesth Analg 2006; 102: 1274-1279.

Roche AM, James MF, Grocott MP, Mythen MG. *Coagulation effects of in vitro serial haemodilution with a balanced electrolyte hetastarch solution compared with a saline-based hetastarch solution and lactated Ringer's solution.* Anaesthesia 2002; 57: 950-957.

Ruttmann TG, James MF, Aronson I. *In vivo investigation into the effects of haemodilution with hydroxyethyl starch (200/0.5) and normal saline on coagulation.* Br J Anaesth 1998; 80: 612-616.

Ruttmann TG, James MF, Viljoen JF. *Haemodilution induces a hypercoagulable state.* Br J Anaesth 1996; 76: 412-414.

Ruttmann TG, James MF, Wells KF. *Effect of 20% in vitro haemodilution with warmed buffered salt solution and cerebrospinal fluid on coagulation.* Br J Anaesth 1999; 82: 110-111.

Schortgen F, Lacherade JC, Bruneel F et al. *Effects of hydroxyethylstarch and gelatin on renal function in severe sepsis: a multicentre randomised study.* Lancet 2001; 357: 911-6.

Schroeder RA, Collins BH, Tuttle-Newhall E et al. *Intraoperative fluid management during orthotopic liver transplantation.* J Cardiothorac Vasc Anesth 2004; 18: 438-41.

Schultz RJ, Whitfield GF, LaMura JJ et al. *The role of physiologic monitoring in patients with fractures of the hip.* Journal of Trauma-Injury Infection & Critical Care 1985; 25: 309-16.

Secher NH and Van Lieshout JJ. *Normovolaemia defined by central blood volume and venous oxygen saturation.* Clin Exp Pharm Physiol 2005; 32: 901-910.

Shires T, Brown FT, Canizaro PC, Summerville N. *Distributional changes in extra cellular fluid during acute hemorrhagic shock.* Surg Forum 1960; 11: 115-117. Abstract not available.

Shires T, Williams J, Brown F. *Acute changes in extracellular fluids associated with major surgical procedures.* Ann Surg 1961; 154: 803-810.

Shoemaker WC, Appel PL, Kram HB et al. *Prospective trial of supranormal values of survivors as therapeutic goals in high-risk surgical patients.* Chest 1988; 94: 1176-86.

Shoemaker WC, Montgomery ES, Kaplan E, and Elwyn DH. *Physiological patterns in surviving and non-surviving shock patients. Use of sequential cardiorespiratory parameters in defining criteria for therapeutic goals and early warning of death.* Archives of Surgery 1973; 106: 630-6. Abstract not available.

Sinclair S, James S, Singer M. *Intraoperative intravascular volume optimisation and length of hospital stay after repair of proximal femoral fracture: randomised controlled trial [see comments].* BMJ 1997; 315: 909-12.

Singer M, De S, V, Vitale D, Jeffcoate W. *Multiorgan failure is an adaptive, endocrine-mediated, metabolic response to overwhelming systemic inflammation.* Lancet 2004 Aug 7; 364(9433): 545-8.

Sjostrand F, Hahn RG: *Volume kinetics of glucose 2.5% solution during laparoscopic cholecystectomy.* Br J Anaesth 2004; 92: 485-92.

Sladen RN, Endo E, Harrison T. *Two-hour versus 22-hour creatinine clearance in critically ill patients.* Anesthesiology 1987; 67: 1013-6. Abstract not available.

Spahn DR, Chassot P-G. CON: *Fluid restriction for cardiac patients during major noncardiac surgery should be replaced by goal-directed intravascular fluid administration.[comment].* Anesthesia & Analgesia 2006; 102: 344-6.

Stump DC, Strauss RG, Henriksen RA, Petersen RE, Saunders R. *Effects of hydroxyethyl starch on blood coagulation, particularly factor VIII.* Transfusion 1985; 25: 349-354.

Svensen C, Hahn RG: *Volume kinetics of Ringer solution, dextran 70, and hypertonic saline in male volunteers.* Anesthesiology 1997; 87: 204-12.

Tabuchi N, de Haan J, Gallandat Huet RC, Boonstra PW, van Oeveren W. *Gelatin use impairs platelet adhesion during cardiac surgery.* Thromb Haemost 1995; 74: 1447-1451.

Tobias MD, Wambold D, Pilla MA, Greer F. *Differential effects of serial hemodilution with hydroxyethyl starch, albumin, and 0.9% saline on whole blood coagulation.* J Clin Anesth 1998; 10: 366-371.

Tocantins LM, Carroll RT, Holburn RH. *The clot accelerating effect of dilution on blood and plasma. Relation to the mechanism of coagulation of normal and hemophiliac blood.* Blood 1951; 6: 720-739. Abstract not available.

Treib J, Haass A, Pindur G, Treib W, Wenzel E, Schimrigk K. *Influence of intravascular molecular weight of hydroxyethyl starch on platelets.* Eur J Haematol 1996; 56: 168-172.

Treib J, Haass A, Pindur G et al. *Increased haemorrhagic risk after repeated infusion of highly substituted medium molecular weight hydroxyethyl starch.* Arzneimittelforschung 1997; 47: 18-22.

Tuchschmidt J, Fried J, Astiz M, Rackow E. *Elevation of cardiac output and oxygen delivery improves outcome in septic shock.* Chest 1992 Jul; 102(1): 216-20.

Tuman KJ, Spiess BD, McCarthy RJ, Ivankovich AD. *Effects of progressive blood loss on coagulation as measured by thrombelastography.* Anesth Analg 1987; 66: 856-863.

Ueno S, Tanabe G, Yamada H, al el. *Response of patients with cirrhosis who have undergone partial hepatectomy to treatment aimed at achieving supranormal oxygen delivery and consumption.* Surgery 1998; 123: 278-86.

Valentine RJ, Duke ML, Inman MH et al. *Effectiveness of pulmonary artery catheters in aortic surgery: a randomized trial.* Journal of Vascular Surgery 1998; 27: 203-11; discussion 211-2.

Van der Linden PJ, De Hert SG, Deraedt D et al. *Hydroxyethyl starch 130/0.4 versus modified fluid gelatin for volume expansion in cardiac surgery patients: the effects on perioperative bleeding and transfusion needs.* Anesth Analg 2005; 101: 629-34.

Venn R, Steele A, Richardson P et al. *Randomized controlled trial to investigate influence of the fluid challenge on duration of hospital stay and perioperative morbidity in patients with hip fractures.* Br J Anaesth 2002; 88: 65-71.

Vogt NH, Bothner U, Lerch G, Lindner KH, Georgieff M. *Large-dose administration of 6% hydroxyethyl starch 200/0.5 total hip arthroplasty: plasma homeostasis, hemostasis, and renal function compared to use of 5% human albumin.* Anesth Analg 1996; 83: 262-268.

von Roten I, Madjdpour C, Frascarolo P et al. *Molar substitution and C2/C6 ratio of hydroxyethyl starch: influence on blood coagulation.* Br J Anaesth 2006; 96: 455-463.

Wakeling HG, McFall MR, Jenkins CS et al. *Intraoperative oesophageal Doppler guided fluid management shortens postoperative hospital stay after major bowel surgery.* Br J Anaesthesia 2005; 95: 634-42.

Wilcox CS. *Regulation of renal blood flow by plasma chloride.* J Clin Invest 1983; 71: 726-35.

Williams EL, Hildebrand KL, McCormick SA, Bedel MJ. *The effect of intravenous lactated Ringer's solution versus 0.9% sodium chloride solution on serum osmolality in human volunteers.* Anesth Analg 1999; 88: 999-1003.

Wilson J, Woods I, Fawcett J, Whall R, Dibb W, Morris C, et al. *Reducing the risk of major elective surgery: randomised controlled trial of preoperative optimisation of oxygen delivery.* BMJ 1999 Apr 24; 318(7191): 1099-103.

Ziegler DW, Wright JG, Choban PS, Flancbaum L. *A prospective randomized trial of preoperative "optimization" of cardiac function in patients undergoing elective peripheral vascular surgery [see comments].* Surgery 1997; 122: 584-92.